Normal Variants and Pitfalls in Musculoskeletal MRI

Guest Editors

WILLIAM B. MORRISON, MD
ADAM C. ZOGA, MD

MAGNETIC RESONANCE IMAGING CLINICS OF NORTH AMERICA

www.mri.theclinics.com

Consulting Editors
VIVIAN S. LEE, MD, PhD, MBA
LYNNE STEINBACH, MD
SURESH MUKHERJI, MD

November 2010 • Volume 18 • Number 4

SAUNDERS an imprint of ELSEVIER, Inc.

W.B. SAUNDERS COMPANY
A Division of Elsevier Inc.

1600 John F. Kennedy Boulevard • Suite 1800 • Philadelphia, Pennsylvania 19103-2899

http://www.theclinics.com

MRI CLINICS OF NORTH AMERICA Volume 18, Number 4
November 2010 ISSN 1064-9689, ISBN 13: 978-1-4557-0303-6

Editor: Joanne Husovski
Developmental Editor: Donald Mumford

Magnetic Resonance Imaging Clinics of North America (ISSN 1064-9689) is published quarterly by Elsevier Inc., 360 Park Avenue South, New York, NY 10010-1710. Months of issue are February, May, August, and November. Business and Editorial Offices: 1600 John F. Kennedy Blvd., Ste. 1800, Philadelphia, PA 19103-2899. Customer Service Office: 3251 Riverport Lane, Maryland Heights, MO 63043. Periodicals postage paid at New York, NY and additional mailing offices. Subscription prices are $309.00 per year (domestic individuals), $501.00 per year (domestic institutions), $158.00 per year (domestic students/residents), $345.00 per year (Canadian individuals), $628.00 per year (Canadian institutions), $448.00 per year (international individuals), $628.00 per year (international institutions), and $228.00 per year (international and Canadian students/residents). International air speed delivery is included in all *Clinics* subscription prices. All prices are subject to change without notice. **POSTMASTER:** Send address changes to *Magnetic Resonance Imaging Clinics*, Elsevier Health Sciences Division, Subscription Customer Service, 3251 Riverport Lane, Maryland Heights, MO 63043. Customer Service (orders, claims, online, change of address): Elsevier Health Sciences Division, Subscription Customer Service, 3251 Riverport Lane, Maryland Heights, MO 63043. Tel:1-800-654-2452 (U.S. and Canada); 314-447-8871 (outside U.S. and Canada). Fax: 314-447-8029. E-mail: journalscustomerservice-usa@elsevier.com (for print support); journalsonlinesupport-usa@elsevier.com (for online support).

Reprints. For copies of 100 or more of articles in this publication, please contact the Commercial Reprints Department, Elsevier Inc., 360 Park Avenue South, New York, NY 10010-1710. Tel.: 212-633-3812; Fax: 212-462-1935; E-mail: reprints@elsevier.com.

Magnetic Resonance Imaging Clinics of North America is covered in the *RSNA Index of Imaging Literature, MEDLINE/PubMed (Index Medicus),* and *EMBASE/Excerpta Medica.*

Printed and bound in the United Kingdom
Transferred to Digital Print 2011

GOAL STATEMENT

The goal of *Magnetic Resonance Imaging Clinics of North America* is to keep practicing physicians up to date with current clinical practice by providing timely articles reviewing the state of the art in patient care.

ACCREDITATION

The *Magnetic Resonance Imaging Clinics of North America* is planned and implemented in accordance with the Essential Areas and Policies of the Accreditation Council for Continuing Medical Education (ACCME) through the joint sponsorship of the University of Virginia School of Medicine and Elsevier. The University of Virginia School of Medicine is accredited by the ACCME to provide continuing medical education for physicians.

The University of Virginia School of Medicine designates this educational activity for a maximum of 15 *AMA PRA Category 1 Credits*™ for each issue, 60 credits per year. Physicians should only claim credit commensurate with the extent of their participation in the activity.

The American Medical Association has determined that physicians not licensed in the US who participate in this CME activity are eligible for a maximum of 15 *AMA PRA Category 1 Credits*™ for each issue, 60 credits per year.

Credit can be earned by reading the text material, taking the CME examination online at http://www.theclinics.com/home/cme, and completing the evaluation. After taking the test, you will be required to review any and all incorrect answers. Following completion of the test and evaluation, your credit will be awarded and you may print your certificate.

FACULTY DISCLOSURE/CONFLICT OF INTEREST

The University of Virginia School of Medicine, as an ACCME accredited provider, endorses and strives to comply with the Accreditation Council for Continuing Medical Education (ACCME) Standards of Commercial Support, Commonwealth of Virginia statutes, University of Virginia policies and procedures, and associated federal and private regulations and guidelines on the need for disclosure and monitoring of proprietary and financial interests that may affect the scientific integrity and balance of content delivered in continuing medical education activities under our auspices.

The University of Virginia School of Medicine requires that all CME activities accredited through this institution be developed independently and be scientifically rigorous, balanced and objective in the presentation/discussion of its content, theories and practices.

All authors/editors participating in an accredited CME activity are expected to disclose to the readers relevant financial relationships with commercial entities occurring within the past 12 months (such as grants or research support, employee, consultant, stock holder, member of speakers bureau, etc.). The University of Virginia School of Medicine will employ appropriate mechanisms to resolve potential conflicts of interest to maintain the standards of fair and balanced education to the reader. Questions about specific strategies can be directed to the Office of Continuing Medical Education, University of Virginia School of Medicine, Charlottesville, Virginia.

The faculty and staff of the University of Virginia Office of Continuing Medical Education have no financial affiliations to disclose.

The authors/editors listed below have identified no professional or financial affiliations for themselves or their spouse/partner:

Fozail Alvi, MD; Jenny T. Bencardino, MD; John A. Carrino, MD, MPH; Eduard de Lange, MD (Test Author); David F. DuBois, MD; Daniel J. Durand, MD; Stephen J. Eustace, MB BCh BAO, MRCPI, FRCR, FFR (RSCI); Darren Fitzpatrick, MD; Soterios Gyftopoulos, MD; Thierry A.G.M. Huisman, MD; Joanne Husovski (Acquisitions Editor); Eoin C. Kavanagh, MB BCh BAO, MRCPI, FFR (RSCI); Joel C. Klena, MD; Vivian S. Lee, MD, PhD, MBA (Consulting Editor); Nancy Major, MD; W. James Malone, DO; Michael R. Moynagh, MB BCh BAO, MRSC; Darra T. Murphy, MB BCh BAO, MRCPI, FFR (RCSI); Imran M. Omar, MD; Marcos Loreto Sampaio, MD; Mark E. Schweitzer, MD; Conor P. Shortt, MB BCh, MSc, FRCR, FFR RCSI; Thomas Slattery, MD; Robert Snowden, MD; Lynne Steinbach, MD (Consulting Editor); Daniel M. Walz, MD; and Adam C. Zoga, MD (Guest Editor).

The authors/editors listed below identified the following professional or financial affiliations for themselves or their spouse/partner:

William B. Morrison, MD (Guest Editor) is a consultant for Apriomed, and is on the Advisory Committee/Board for GE (ONI).
Suresh Mukherji, MD (Consulting Editor) is a consultant for Philips.

Disclosure of Discussion of non-FDA approved uses for pharmaceutical products and/or medical devices:
The University of Virginia School of Medicine, as an ACCME provider, requires that all faculty presenters identify and disclose any "off label" uses for pharmaceutical and medical device products. The University of Virginia School of Medicine recommends that each physician fully review all the available data on new products or procedures prior to instituting them with patients.

TO ENROLL

To enroll in the Magnetic Resonance Imaging Clinics of North America Continuing Medical Education program, call customer service at 1-800-654-2452 or visit us online at www.theclinics.com/home/cme. The CME program is available to subscribers for an additional fee of $196.00.

Contributors

CONSULTING EDITORS

VIVIAN S. LEE, MD, PhD, MBA
Professor of Radiology, Physiology, and
Neurosciences; Vice-Dean for Science; and
Senior Vice-President and Chief Scientific
Officer at New York University Langone
Medical Center, New York, New York

LYNNE STEINBACH, MD
Professor of Clinical Radiology and Orthopaedic
Surgery at the University of California San
Francisco, San Francisco, California

SURESH MUKHERJI, MD
Professor and Chief of Neuroradiology
and Head and Neck Radiology;
Professor of Radiology, Otolaryngology
Head Neck Surgery, Radiation Oncology,
Oral Medicine, and Periodontics
at the University of Michigan Health System,
Ann Arbor, Michigan

GUEST EDITORS

WILLIAM B. MORRISON, MD
Professor of Radiology; Chief of
Musculoskeletal Radiology, Thomas Jefferson
University Hospital, Philadelphia, Pennsylvania

ADAM C. ZOGA, MD
Associate Professor of Radiology; Director
of Musculoskeletal MRI, Thomas Jefferson
University Hospital, Philadelphia, Pennsylvania

AUTHORS

FOZAIL ALVI, MD
Department of Radiology, Geisinger Medical
Center, Danville, Pennsylvania

JENNY T. BENCARDINO, MD
Associate Professor, Department of Radiology,
New York University Hospital for Joint
Diseases, New York, New York

JOHN A. CARRINO, MD, MPH
Russell H. Morgan Department of Radiology
and Radiological Science; Associate Professor
of Radiology; Section Chief, Division of
Musculoskeletal Radiology, Johns Hopkins
Medical Institutions, Baltimore, Maryland

DAVID F. DUBOIS, MD
Department of Radiology, Northwestern
University Feinberg School of Medicine,
Chicago, Illinois

DANIEL J. DURAND, MD
Russell H. Morgan Department of Radiology
and Radiological Science, Division of
Musculoskeletal Radiology, Johns Hopkins
Medical Institutions, Baltimore, Maryland

**STEPHEN J. EUSTACE, MB BCh BAO,
MRCPI, FRCR, FFR (RSCI)**
Professor, Department of Radiology, Mater
Misericordiae University Hospital; Department
of Radiology, Cappagh National Orthopaedic
Hospital, Finglas, Dublin, Ireland

DARREN FITZPATRICK, MD
Department of Radiology, North Shore
University Hospital, Manhasset, New York

SOTERIOS GYFTOPOULOS, MD
Clinical Fellow in Musculoskeletal Radiology,
Department of Radiology, New York University
Hospital for Joint Diseases, New York,
New York

THIERRY A.G.M. HUISMAN, MD
Russell H. Morgan Department of Radiology
and Radiological Science; Medical Director
and Professor, Division of Pediatric Radiology,
Johns Hopkins Medical Institutions, Baltimore,
Maryland

EOIN C. KAVANAGH, MB BCh BAO, MRCPI, FFR (RSCI)
Department of Radiology, Mater Misericordiae University Hospital, Dublin, Ireland

JOEL C. KLENA, MD
Department of Orthopedic Surgery, Geisinger Medical Center, Danville, Pennsylvania

NANCY MAJOR, MD
Professor of Radiology and Orthopaedics; Chief, Musculoskeletal Radiology, Department of Radiology, Hospital of the University of Pennsylvania, Philadelphia, Pennsylvania

W. JAMES MALONE, DO
Director Musculoskeletal Imaging, Department of Radiology, Geisinger Medical Center, Danville, Pennsylvania

MICHAEL R. MOYNAGH, MB BCh BAO, MRSC
Department of Radiology, Mater Misericordiae University Hospital, Dublin, Ireland

DARRA T. MURPHY, MB BCh BAO, MRCPI, FFR (RCSI)
Department of Radiology, Mater Misericordiae University Hospital; Department of Radiology, Cappagh National Orthopaedic Hospital, Finglas, Dublin, Ireland

IMRAN M. OMAR, MD
Department of Radiology, Northwestern University Feinberg School of Medicine, Chicago, Illinois

MARCOS LORETO SAMPAIO, MD
Assistant of the Musculoskeletal Radiology Department, The Ottawa Hospital, University of Ottawa, Ottawa, Ontario, Canada

MARK E. SCHWEITZER, MD
Chief of the Radiology Department, The Ottawa Hospital; Chief of Diagnostic Imaging and Full Professor, University of Ottawa, Ottawa, Ontario, Canada

CONOR P. SHORTT, MB BCh, MSc, FRCR, FFR RCSI
Assistant Professor of Radiology, Department of Radiology, Thomas Jefferson University Hospital, Philadelphia, Pennsylvania

THOMAS SLATTERY, MD
Department of Radiology, Pennsylvania Hospital of the University of Pennsylvania Health System, Philadelphia, Pennsylvania

ROBERT SNOWDEN, MD
Department of Radiology, Geisinger Medical Center, Danville, Pennsylvania

DANIEL M. WALZ, MD
Assistant Professor of Radiology, Division of Musculoskeletal Imaging, Department of Radiology, North Shore University Hospital, Hofstra University School of Medicine, Manhasset, New York

Contents

> The appearance of osseous, labral, hyaline cartilage, ligament, muscle, and tendon variants and pitfalls are discussed with attention to the keys to distinguishing each of the findings from pathologic lesions of the shoulder.

> Imaging variants of the elbow and pitfalls can be disconcerting and can lead to diagnostic mistakes. Inhomogeneities in the magnetic field and coil position can result in signal changes that may simulate abnormality. Bone signal and morphology variants, such as the islands of red marrow and the pseudodefect of the capitellum and intraarticular inclusions such as plicae, may be mistaken for abnormal findings. Variations of the distal biceps and triceps tendons and different aspects of the ligaments and their insertions, as well as nonpathologic signal and width changes in the ulnar nerve, are other examples of common pitfalls in magnetic resonance imaging of the elbow.

> The radiologist serves as an indispensable consultant for those patients with wrist pain, by determining the causes of the pain and severity of the injury, helping to determine treatment options, and providing preoperative guidance for surgery, if planned. This article reviews normal anatomic variants and potential danger areas encountered by the radiologist when interpreting magnetic resonance imaging of the wrist.

> MR imaging of the hip is one of the most common musculoskeletal MR imaging studies performed today to assess for occult fractures, acetabular labral tears, hyaline cartilage loss, and musculotendinous injuries. Several developmental variations are seen in the hip, which can be mistaken for disease or potentially even contribute to the development of a pathologic condition. As in any imaging study, it is important to be cognizant of these variations as well as associated findings that help distinguish between true abnormality and developmental variation when interpreting an MR image of the hip. This article describes the numerous variants of the hip that are frequently seen on arthrographic and nonarthrographic MR imaging examinations.

Magnetic Resonance Imaging Clinics of North America

THE CLINICS ARE NOW AVAILABLE ONLINE!

Access your subscription at:
www.theclinics.com

Preface
Normal Variants and Pitfalls in Musculoskeletal MRI

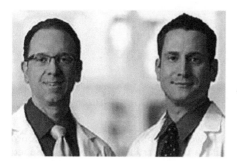

William B. Morrison, MD   Adam C. Zoga, MD
Guest Editors

For radiologists, the term "normal variant" is introduced during the very early stages of training, perhaps even on the first day of residency. Seeing an azygous lobe for the first time seemed innocuous enough, but things got a bit more nerve-wracking during the first week of night float when a child in the E.D. had focal tenderness at a fragmented apophysis that looked just like in image in the Keats normal variants reference book. Indeed, it is difficult to confidently use the word "normal" in a report when an anatomic structure just doesn't look right on radiography, CT, MRI, ultrasound, or even scintigraphy or PET imaging. The human body is rife with potential imaging pitfalls. It is essential for imagers to draw upon a knowledge base of anatomic structures that vary from the routine in their imaging appearance, but still fall within the realm of normal anatomy. With increasing imaging options, image resolution, and overall understanding of physiologic biomechanics, the musculoskeletal system abounds with normal imaging variants and pitfalls, both old and new. It is also essential for even seasoned, expert radiologists to have access to a reference where guidance can be sought when something just doesn't look right, but it is not clearly pathologic and may reflect a variant of normal anatomy. We hope that this volume can fill the role of such a reference for MRI of the musculoskeletal system (**Fig. 1**).

What is normal? It is curious how terms like "within normal limits" are rarely taught to first year residents during side-by-side workstation readouts, but then creep into trainee reports with increasing frequency once the resident or fellow is previewing dictating on his or her own, as in the setting of night float. This phenomenon reflects an underlying uncertainty about the limits of normal variation experienced to some degree by all physicians interpreting imaging studies, even veteran subspecialty radiologists. As imaging evolves, so does our understanding of normal imaging appearances, and few arenas within the radiologic sciences have evolved more rapidly and significantly over the past 15 years than MRI of the musculoskeletal system. Some imaging findings once considered to be normal variants are now accepted to be indicators or at least associates of well-published musculoskeletal injuries. Cystic change at the greater tuberosity of the humerus was often disregarded as normal variation, before an association between these cysts and rotator cuff tendinopathy was published.[1] Other reproducible imaging findings previously categorized as pathology are now accepted as normal anatomic structures and are potential pitfalls in imaging interpretation. Many articular cartilage defects were erroneously reported at the posterior margin of the capitellum in the elbow before the pseudodefect was described as

Magn Reson Imaging Clin N Am 18 (2010) xi–xiii
doi:10.1016/j.mric.2010.11.001

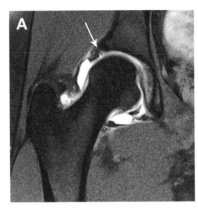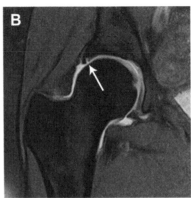

Fig. 1. (A, B) Is this a normal variant, a pitfall, or a pathologic lesion? Two different patients with clinical concern for acetabular labrum tear show similar clefts between the acetabular articular cartilage and the anterosuperior acetabular labrum (*arrows*). One was called a normal variant (A) and one was called a labral tear (B). An argument can be made for either diagnosis in both cases based on the current musculoskeletal imaging literature. The enclosed chapters discuss this and other similar conundra throughout musculoskeletal system.

a normal variant in the imaging literature.[2] Another group of anatomic nuances remain controversial, with some scientific publications and authors describing them as normal variants and others describing them as pathologic lesions. The possibility of a normal sublabral recess within the acetabular labrum remains a hot button issue, while the perilabral recess and the stellate crease have become almost unanimously accepted as normal hip variants.[3,4]

This is an issue of *Magnetic Resonance Imaging Clinics* that will require incremental updates, but we have aligned a group of authors with tremendous experience and insight into both the science and the art of MRI of the musculoskeletal system. Each article reviews up-to-date science as well as explores and discusses controversial issues. The glenohumeral joint is rife with anatomic idiosyncrasies, and Drs Fitzpatrick and Walz from North Shore Hospital in New York detail the current state of shoulder variants. Drs Sampaio and Schweitzer from the University of Ottawa update us on elbow variants on MRI, and Dr Jamie Malone and his colleagues from Geisinger Medical Center cover the wrist and hand. Turning to the lower extremity, Dr DuBois and Omar from Northwestern University Medical Center review the rapidly accumulating literature on hip MRI, and Drs Slattery and Major from the University of Pennsylvania outline the many nuances of knee MRI anatomy. Then, Drs Gyftopoulos and Bencardino from New York University cover the ankle and our colleague Conor Shortt from Thomas Jefferson handles the midfoot and forefoot. The axial skeleton has its own set of variants, and Drs Durand, Huisman, and Carrino from Johns Hopkins University update us on the various regions of the spine, while

Drs Murphy, Kavanagh, and their colleagues from the Mater Misericordiae in Dublin, Ireland provide guidelines for assessing bone marrow on MRI.

Surgical and arthroscopic techniques continue to evolve as imaging improves, and it is imperative for imagers to work together with surgeons to establish which of these pits, cysts, bumps, and morphologic aberrancies can be firmly categorized as true normal variants, and which might be precursors or ramifications of disease. As new findings are observed at imaging and in the operating room, we must continue to retrospectively review our imaging vault to see if we are discovering new pathologic lesions, or simply additional idiosyncrasies of musculoskeletal anatomy. The term "normal variation" is a moving target, and there will always be new imaging findings to explore. We hope that this issue of *MRI Clinics* will serve as a reference for accepted imaging pitfalls as well as a building block for progressive work in the identification, description, and proper categorization of observations as pathology or normal variation.

William B. Morrison, MD
Thomas Jefferson University Hospital
132 South 10th Street, 1079A
Philadelphia, PA 19107, USA

Adam C. Zoga, MD
Thomas Jefferson University Hospital
132 South 10th Street, 1083A
Philadelphia, PA 19107, USA

E-mail addresses:
william.morrison@jefferson.edu (W.B. Morrison)
adam.zoga@jefferson.edu (A.C. Zoga)

REFERENCES

1. Fritz LB, Ouellette HA, O'Hanley TA, et al. Cystic changes at supraspinatus and infraspinatus tendon insertion sites: association with age and rotator cuff disorders in 238 patients. Radiology 2007;244(1): 239–48.

2. Rosenberg ZS, Beltran J, Cheung Y, et al. MR imaging of the elbow: normal variant and potential diagnostic pitfalls of the trochlear groove and cubital tunnel. AJR Am J Roentgenol 1995;164(2): 415–8.

3. Studler U, Kalberer F, Leunig M, et al. MR arthrography of the hip: differentiation between an anterior sublabral recess as a normal variant and a labral tear. Radiology 2008;249(3):947–54.

4. Zoga AC. Hip labrum tear. In: Sonin A, Manaster BJ, et al, editors. Diagnostic imaging: Musculoskeletal trauma. Salt Lake City (UT): Amirsys; 2010. p. 5, 80–5.

Shoulder MR Imaging Normal Variants and Imaging Artifacts

Darren Fitzpatrick, MD[a], Daniel M. Walz, MD[b],*

KEYWORDS

• Normal variants • Imaging artifacts • Shoulder MR Imaging

MR imaging of the shoulder is commonly used to evaluate patients with shoulder impingement, acute and chronic rotator cuff pathology, and instability lesions. Interpreting radiologists, therefore, need to apply knowledge not only of the imaging appearance of these pathologic conditions but also of normal anatomic variants and imaging artifacts. The ability to discern these findings from true pathology is essential in providing a useful and accurate interpretation for referring clinicians. The appearance of osseous, labral, hyaline cartilage, ligament, muscle, and tendon variants and pitfalls is discussed with attention to the keys to distinguishing each of the findings from pathologic lesions of the shoulder.

OSSEOUS STRUCTURES
Acromion

The acromion process has been classified into different types based on shape. Bigliani and colleagues[1] first described three types based on the undersurface morphology:

> Type 1: straight or flat
> Type 2: curved
> Type 3: hooked.

Since this initial description, a fourth type has been added describing a convex or upward pointing undersurface.

These acromial morphologic variations were initially described by using scapular Y-view radiographs; however, they also can be accurately characterized on shoulder MR imaging using sagittal oblique and coronal oblique sequences (**Fig. 1**).[2]

The association of differing acromial morphology with subacromial impingement and rotator cuff disease has been disputed. Some investigators think that a type 3 acromion is developmental in origin from traction of the coracoacromial ligament, creating an enthesophyte,[3] whereas others consider it a morphologic variant. In either case, a type 3 acromion or prominent enthesophyte can play a primary role in subacromial impingement syndrome[1] and in injury to the anterior leading edge of the supraspinatus. Other morphologic changes, such as a downward-projecting keel spur from the acromion (**Fig. 2**) or lateral downsloping of the acromion (**Fig. 3**), also likely result in the development of rotator cuff pathology.[4] Although disputed, the relationship between acromial morphology and subacromial impingement remains an often applied rationale for subacromial decompression surgery in patients with rotator cuff pathology.

The acromion is formed by multiple ossification centers, one that appears at 3 months of fetal life and others that follow during later teenage years. Embryologically, the acromion is divided into the basiacromion, meta-acromion, mesoacromion, and preacromion (**Fig. 4**). After age 25 years, nonfusion of these ossification centers can result in formation of an accessory ossicle, or os acromiale. This is found in up to 15% of shoulders and, when present, is bilateral in one-third of cases.[5,6] Multiple shapes and sizes of the os acromiale are possible based on the site of fusion failure.[7] An

[a] Department of Radiology, North Shore University Hospital, 300 Community Drive, Manhasset, NY 11030, USA
[b] Division of Musculoskeletal Imaging, Department of Radiology, North Shore University Hospital, Hofstra University School of Medicine, 300 Community Drive, Manhasset, NY 11030, USA
* Corresponding author.
E-mail address: danwalz@hotmail.com

Magn Reson Imaging Clin N Am 18 (2010) 615–632
doi:10.1016/j.mric.2010.07.006

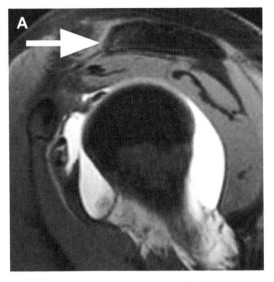
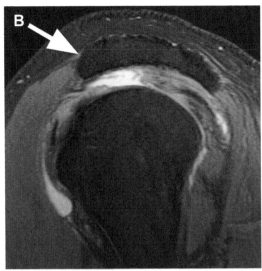
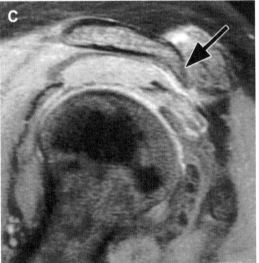

Fig. 1. Acromion shapes. Sagittal oblique T1-weighted fat-suppressed images demonstrate (*A*) flat type 1 acromion (*arrow*) and (*B*) curved type 2 acromion (*arrow*). (*C*) Sagittal oblique PD-weighted fat-suppressed image from an MR arthrogram demonstrates the hooked morphology of a type 3 acromion (*arrow*).

os acromiale is best identified on axial MR images, where a signal gap is seen between the fat-containing marrow of the distal acromion and the nonfused os (**Fig. 5**). The os forms a pseudoarticulation with the base of the acromion via fibrous tissue, periosteum, cartilage, or synovium accounting for the variability seen on T2-weighted images. On sagittal MR imaging, the presence of the os can be determined because it is the site of attachment of the coracoacromial ligament, which inserts on its anterior-inferior border. The presence of a double acromioclavicular joint may be seen on sagittal images, where the os is seen articulating with both the native acromion and the clavicle. It is important to identify

an os acromiale because it may play a role in the development of shoulder impingement symptoms due to inferior displacement with deltoid contraction. Its presence may also serve as a contraindication to subacromial decompression surgery in cases of clinical shoulder impingement. Equally important is that degenerative changes across the synchondrosis or associated acromioclavicular degeneration may be an isolated source of shoulder pain (**Fig. 6**).[3]

Humerus

The proximal humerus, including the head, greater and lesser tuberosities, and anatomic neck, all

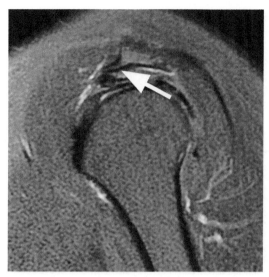

Fig. 2. Acromial keel spur. Sagittal oblique PD-weighted fat-suppressed image demonstrates a large downward-projecting acromial spur (*arrow*) resembling the keel of a sailboat.

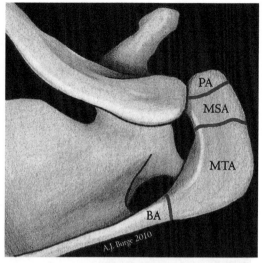

Fig. 4. Illustration of the acromion ossification centers. BA, basiacromion; MSA, mesoacromion; MTA, meta-acromion; PA, preacromion. (*Courtesy of Alissa J. Burge, MD.*)

contribute to the articulation of the glenohumeral joint. The bicipital or intertubercular groove, located between the greater and lesser tuberosities, contains the extra-articular long head of the biceps tendon at the anterior aspect of the humerus. An additional, normal groove exists at the posterior aspect of the humerus near the junction of the head and proximal diaphysis (**Fig. 7**).

This is a potential source of a false-positive interpretation on axial MR imaging and should not be mistaken for a Hill-Sachs lesion, a posterolateral impaction fracture of the humeral head as a result of anterior shoulder dislocation (**Fig. 8**). This distinction becomes important in patients with a history of glenohumeral dislocation, because the presence of a Hill-Sachs lesion may warrant further surgical treatment in addition to repair of the anterior-inferior glenoid and labrum. There

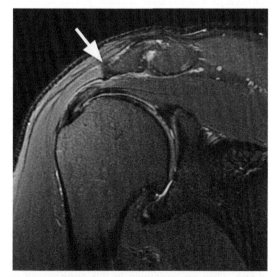

Fig. 3. Lateral downsloping acromion. Coronal oblique PD-weighted fat-suppressed image in a patient with clinical subacromial impingement shows lateral downsloping of the acromion (*arrow*) narrowing the subacromial space.

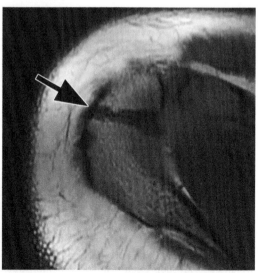

Fig. 5. Os acromiale. Axial PD-weighted image demonstrates an os acromiale with a low-signal gap at the mesoacromion ossification center (*arrow*).

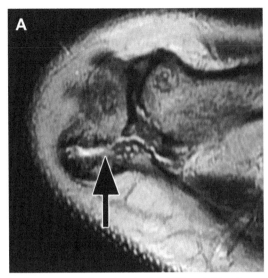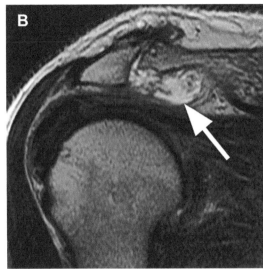

Fig. 6. Os acromiale arthrosis. Axial PD-weighted image (*A*) demonstrates an os acromiale with marked degeneration and fluid signal at the snychondrosis (*black arrow*). Coronal oblique PD-weighted (*B*) image demonstrates extension of this fluid signal inferior to the acromioclavicular joint with synovial debris consistent with synovitis (*white arrow*).

can be overlap in the appearance of a normal posterolateral humeral groove and a Hill-Sachs lesion, although delineation of the two can be determined by their location within the humerus. Hill-Sachs lesions are visible on the uppermost axial sections of the humerus and are positioned within 5 mm of the top of the humeral head superolaterally. The normal anatomic groove of the humerus usually lies 20 to 30 mm from the superior

Fig. 7. Normal posterior humeral groove. Axial PD-weighted fat-suppressed image demonstrates a normal groove (*arrow*) at the posterior aspect of the humeral head. This is both more medial and inferior when compared with a Hill-Sachs lesion.

humeral head and is positioned more posteriorly and medial on axial sections. The depth and width of the posterolateral defect are not reliable indicators to its origin.[8]

Glenoid

The glenoid cavity is the site of articulation of the scapula with the humeral head. Its lack of depth provides increased range of motion of the glenohumeral joint at the cost of stability. This is, therefore, provided by the surrounding structures, in particular the glenohumeral ligaments, labrum, and rotator cuff. Various imaging abnormalities and variations of the glenoid may be present. At the midpoint of the circle defined by the anterior, posterior, superior, and inferior borders of the glenoid, there is an area of thickened subchondral bone with thinned overlying cartilage (**Fig. 9**). This osseous prominence is termed *the tubercle of Ossaki* and should not be mistaken for an area of cartilaginous thinning or loss. Similarly, in this same area, a smooth, benign-appearing, full-thickness cartilage defect without thickened underlying bone can be seen as a normal variant (**Fig. 10**), not to be mistaken for chondromalacia.[6]

The shape of the articulating osseous glenoid as seen in the oblique sagittal plane can be round, ovoid, teardrop-shaped, or pear-shaped. The shape relies on variations in the appearance of the glenoid notch, which can be prominent, diminutive, or absent. The glenoid notch lies at the anterior margin of the glenoid at its upper one-third margin and accounts for the often pear-shaped

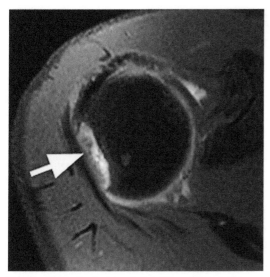

Fig. 8. Hill-Sachs lesion. Axial PD-weighted fat-suppressed image demonstrates a large superolateral impaction fracture of the humerus (*arrow*) in a patient status post anterior dislocation.

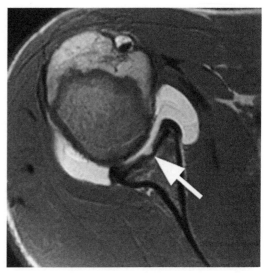

Fig. 10. Benign glenoid cartilage defect. Axial PD-weighted image from an MR arthrogram demonstrates a smooth, central, full-thickness region of cartilage absence (*arrow*) that is a normal variant and should not be mistaken for grade 4 chondromalacia.

appearance of the glenoid on sagittal images (**Fig. 11**). An oval glenoid on sagittal images is produced by the absence of a glenoid notch. The labrum is not attached to the bony margin of the glenoid at the notch, resulting in the sublabral recess.[9] Observation of an inverted pear shape (or a bite taken from the pear) on sagittal images is an important distinction because this

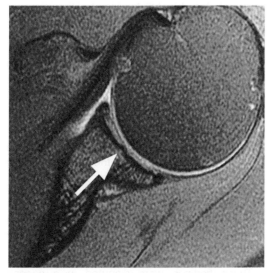

Fig. 9. Tubercle of Ossaki. Axial PD-weighted fat-suppressed image demonstrates a focal area of thickened subchondral bone (*arrow*) with thinned overlying hyaline cartilage in the geometric center of the glenoid.

morphology is indicative of the presence of an osseous Bankart lesion (**Fig. 12**).

Inui and colleagues[10] evaluated glenoid version using 3-D MR imaging and demonstrated a change in tilt from posterior to anterior when evaluating the glenoid in axial plane from superior to inferior. Similarly, they showed that the glenoid cavity was most often (82.5%) concave inferiorly and rarely (7.5%) concave superiorly (**Fig. 13**). This morphology explains external rotation of the upper extremity with arm elevation. This creates two distinct surfaces of the glenoid with the superior aspect directed posteriorly with a small angle of curvature receiving the humeral head when the arm is raised. In contradistinction, the inferior glenoid, angled anteriorly with a small radius of curvature, receives the humeral head when the arm is lowered.

The posterior rim of the glenoid can also vary in shape and configuration. Three morphologic shapes of the posterior glenoid rim predominate: pointed (normal), rounded (lazy J), and triangular-shaped osseous deficiency (delta).[11] The lazy J and delta shapes have been implicated in posterior (atraumatic) shoulder joint instability.[12] Distinguishing between the shapes of the posterior labrum can sometimes be challenging on MR imaging because the low signal of the cortex blends in with fibrous low signal of the posterior labrum. Glenoid hypoplasia/dysplasia represents an extreme of the spectrum of posterior glenoid abnormalities. Affected patients present with

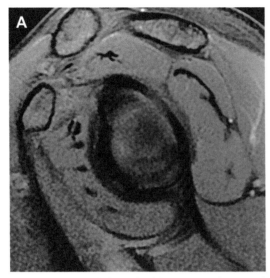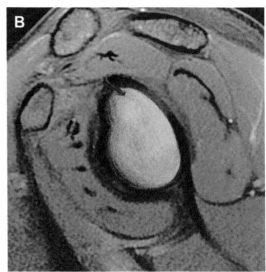

Fig. 11. Pear-shaped glenoid. Oblique sagittal PD weighted fat-suppressed image (*A*) and same image with super-imposed pear (*B*) illustration demonstrate the pear shape of the glenoid cavity created by the presence of the glenoid notch anterosuperiorly. (*Courtesy of* Alissa J. Burge, MD.)

posterior or multidirectional instability. This entity has typical features on MR imaging, including an irregular articular surface, a notched inferior rim of the glenoid with corresponding hypoplasia of the scapular neck, and humeral head along with a bulbous, hypertrophied posterior labrum (**Fig. 14**). The humeral head is usually subluxed posteriorly.[6]

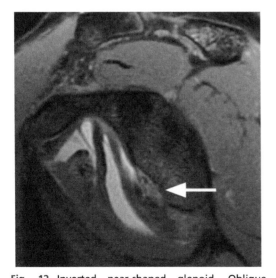

Fig. 12. Inverted pear-shaped glenoid. Oblique sagittal PD-weighted fat-suppressed image of the shoulder demonstrates an osseous defect (*arrow*) at the anteroinferior glenoid consistent with a Bankart lesion.

TENDONS
Long Head of the Biceps Brachii

The intra-articular portion of the long head of the biceps originates from the supraglenoid tuberosity and/or the superior labrum (biceps-labral complex or biceps anchor), to varying degrees. Although the origin was initially thought primarily an osseous attachment, in cadaveric studies, a majority of shoulders demonstrated a predominant attachment of the biceps tendon to the superior labrum.[13] The attachment of the tendon to the superior labrum also varies, however, with contributions from both its anterior and posterior aspects (**Fig. 15**). In the gross dissection of 100 shoulders, the distribution of the origin of the biceps tendon relative to the superior labrum was as follows[14]:

1. Posterior labrum only (22%)
2. Predominately from the posterior labrum with small attachment site to the anterior labrum (33%)
3. Equal origins from the anterior and posterior labrum (37%)
4. Predominately from the anterior labrum with small attachment site to the posterior labrum (8%).

These findings were disputed in a second cadaveric study where the variations in the distribution of biceps attachment to the superior labrum were determined to be based on variations in the insertion of the IGHL.[15] Additional reports have

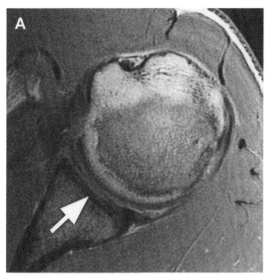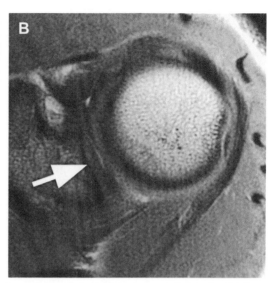

Fig. 13. Glenoid version. (*A*) Axial PD-weighted image through the more inferior aspect of the glenoid shows a concave shape with slight anterior version (*arrow*). (*B*) Axial image through the superior glenoid in the same patient shows a flat shape with posterior version (*arrow*).

shown portions of the biceps tendon attaching to the capsule itself or the rotator cuff.[16,17]

In addition to the location of the biceps attachment to the superior labrum, there is variation in the morphology of the biceps-labral complex (**Fig. 16**). A type 1 biceps-labral complex attaches firmly to the superior glenoid. When a type II complex is present, a small sublabral sulcus is present that may communicate with a sublabral

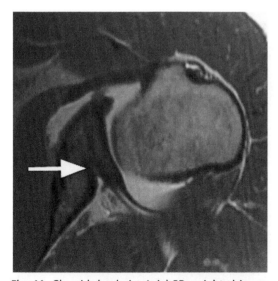

Fig. 14. Glenoid dysplasia. Axial PD-weighted image from an MR arthrogram demonstrates marked hypoplasia of the posterior osseous glenoid (*arrow*) and an associated hypertrophied irregular-appearing posterior labrum.

hole. A type III complex has a meniscus-shaped labrum with a large sulcus.[18] Predominately posterior attachments also display a large recess resulting in a more mobile biceps-labral complex.[6]

From the scapular and labral attachment, the biceps travels through the joint into the rotator interval where it is intracapsular but extrasynovial. Possible imaging pitfalls of the intracapsular long biceps tendon include intermediate signal intensity throughout the normally low-signal tendon as it courses anteriorly in the joint due to magic angle artifact (**Fig. 17**). Also, as the intra-articular portion of the tendon courses superiorly and posteriorly from the bicipital groove to the biceps anchor, it can appear displaced medially, mimicking medial dislocation of the tendon (**Fig. 18**). Fibers of portions of the coracohumeral ligament, the superior glenohumeral ligament, and the superior-most fibers of the supraspinatus form a sling around the intra-articular biceps tendon proximal to the bicipital groove, called the biceps pulley. The tendon then courses anteriorly into the bicipital groove, between the greater and lesser tuberosities, where it is stabilized by a structure, termed *the transverse humeral ligament*. This is formed by contributions of fibers from the supraspinatus, subscapularis, coracohumeral ligament, and the joint capsule. Within the bicipital groove, normal structures that are seen to varying degrees include the biceps vincula (synovial bands attaching to the biceps within the tendon sheath) (**Fig. 19**), blood vessels, a duplicated or bifed long head of the biceps, or anterior, leading-edge fibers of the supraspinatus ectopically inserting within the groove (**Fig. 20**).

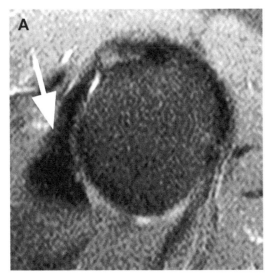
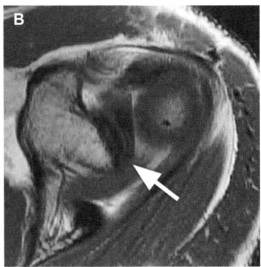

Fig. 15. Biceps-labral junction. (A) Axial PD-weighted fat-suppressed image of the shoulder shows a far anterior attachment of the biceps to the superior labrum (arrow). (B) Axial PD-weighted image in a different patient demonstrates a far posterior attachment (arrow).

Rotator Cuff

Magic angle effect is a physical phenomenon that occurs due to orientation of tendon fibers at 55° relative to the main magnetic field.[19] Tendons are composed primarily of collagen, which is anisotropic, causing T2 relaxation properties to vary with the angle of measurement.[20] At the magic angle of 55°, the T2 of the collagen-containing tendon is increased. This effect on signal is minimal when the echo time (TE) is long. On short TE sequences (T1 and intermediate-weighted/proton density [PD]), however, the tendon appears increased in signal, mimicking the appearance of tendinosis or partial tendon tearing. The area of signal abnormality within the tendon does not persist or is diminished on longer TE sequences (T2-weighted images), necessitating the use of such sequences to distinguished magic angle

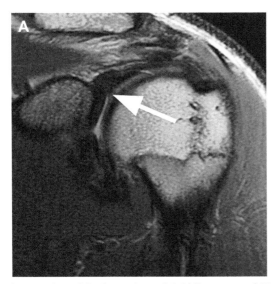
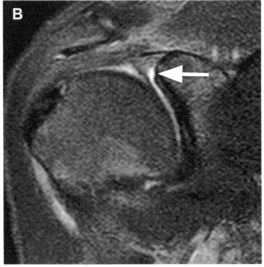

Fig. 16. Biceps-labral complexes. (A) Oblique coronal PD-weighted image demonstrates a firm attachment of the labrum (arrow) to the glenoid at the level of the biceps anchor consistent with a type 1 biceps-labral complex. (B) Coronal oblique PD-weighted fat-suppressed image in a different patient shows a prominent fluid-filled sulcus (arrow) consistent with a type 3 complex.

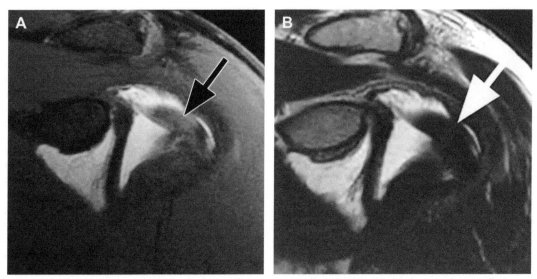

Fig. 17. Biceps magic angle artifact. Oblique coronal T1-weighted (*A*) and T2-weighted (*B*) images of the shoulder demonstrate diffuse intermediate signal within the intra-articular biceps (*black arrow*) with a TE of 10. This signal resolves (*white arrow*) on the T2-weighted image with a TE of 100.

artifact from rotator cuff tendinosis or partial tendon tearing (**Fig. 21**).[21]

Although occasionally difficult to identify on MR imaging (easier on MR arthrography), there is a sulcus of uncovered bone between the osseous insertion of the supraspinatus and the articular cartilage (**Fig. 22**).[22] Knowing the fixed width (1.5 to 2.0 mm) of this sulcus, arthroscopists can determine the amount of tendon loss in partial thickness articular surface tears. The presence of this sulcus is important because this small area of exposed bone should not be mistaken for a small, articular surface tear and the size of articular surface tears should be measured with knowledge of the typical

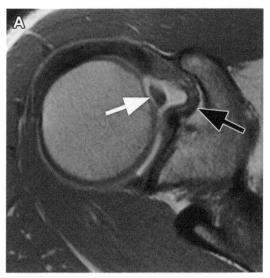
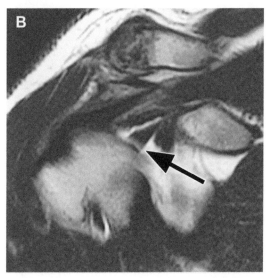

Fig. 18. Pseudosubluxation of the biceps tendon. (*A*) Axial PD-weighted image from an MR arthrogram demonstrates apparent medial subluxation (*white arrow*). (*B*) The oblique coronal T2-weighted image confirms the presence of the long head of the biceps within the bicipital groove then taking a sharp turn within the joint (*black arrow*) related to anatomic variation and slight internal rotation. The SGHL is seen arising from the anterosuperior labrum (*black arrow* in [*A*]).

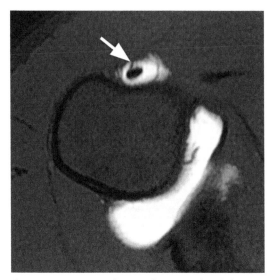

Fig. 19. Biceps vincula. Axial T1-weighted fat-suppressed image from an MR arthrogram demonstrates a thin low-signal band within the biceps tendon sheath attaching to the long head of the biceps tendon consistent with the biceps vincula (*arrow*).

size of this sulcus so as to not overestimate the degree of tearing. Widening of the sulcus may indicate regression of the articular cartilage or partial undersurface tearing.[23]

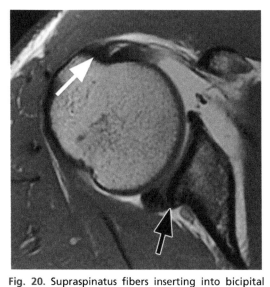

Fig. 20. Supraspinatus fibers inserting into bicipital groove. Axial PD-weighted image from an MR arthrogram demonstrates the anterior edge of the supraspinatus inserting into the superior aspect of the bicipital groove (*white arrow*). Note the lazy J configuration of the posterior glenoid and hypertrophied labrum (*black arrow*) in this patient with mild glenoid dysplasia.

GLENOHUMERAL LIGAMENT AND CAPSULAR VARIANTS
Inferior Glenohumeral Ligament

The largest glenohumeral ligament, the inferior glenohumeral ligament (IGHL), is the main stabilizing ligament of the shoulder, supporting the humerus in external and internal rotation during abduction.[3] The ligament consists of anterior and posterior bands with the intervening axillary recess of the joint capsule. The IGHL is almost invariably present and, when not directly visualized on MR arthrography, it is usually present as a thickening of the joint capsule.[6]

The anterior band of the IGHL may insert proximally on the anterior labrum between the 2-o'clock and 4-o'clock locations, just medial to the labrum on the glenoid, or more proximally on the scapular neck. This variation causes differences in the size of the subscapularis recess,[3] which also varies in size based on the position of the shoulder.

The posterior band of the IGHL is usually smaller and inserts at approximately the 9-o'clock position of the labrum, more medially along the glenoid, or on the posterior aspect of the scapular neck (**Fig. 23**). Both bands of the IGHL and the intervening axillary pouch insert on the humeral neck. The intervening insertion of the axillary recess on the humeral neck may create a jagged or corrugated appearance on MR arthrography.[24] Thickening of the IGHL and the axillary pouch is a nonspecific finding but can be seen in patients with adhesive capsulitis (**Fig. 24**).

Middle Glenohumeral Ligament

The middle glenohumeral ligament (MGHL) serves to stabilize the shoulder in abduction and shows the greatest variation of all the glenohumeral ligaments. The MGHL may attach to the anterosuperior labrum (usually just below the origin of the superior glenohumeral ligament) or attach to the anterior scapular neck itself, where it may simulate capsular disruption associated with anterior instability (**Fig. 25**). The MGHL may have a conjoined insertion with the superior glenohumeral ligament or the IGHL (see **Fig. 25**). It may also have a common insertion with the long head of the biceps tendon, particularly in cases where the superior glenohumeral ligament is absent. The size of the MGHL may be variable; it may be diminutive or thickened and cord-like.[25] The MGHL is most prominent in the Buford complex, where the anterosuperior labrum is absent with compensatory thickening of the MGHL (**Fig. 26**). This occurs in 1.5% of shoulders.[26,27] The Buford complex is important to recognize because it may simulate detachment of the anterior superior labrum.

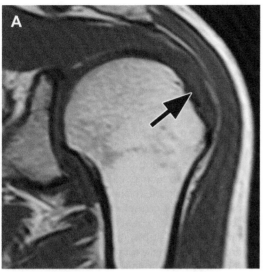
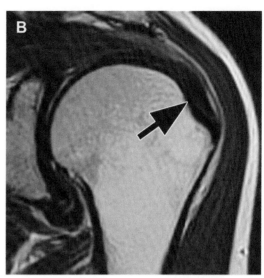

Fig. 21. Rotator cuff magic angle artifact. Coronal T1- and T2-weighted images through the supraspinatus insertion demonstrate increased (*A*) intermediate signal on the short TE sequence (*arrow*) that is not seen on the (*B*) longer TE sequence (*arrow*).

Additionally, the MGHL may be duplicated, which must be distinguished from a type VII SLAP lesion.[6] The MGHL may be redundant or infolded or may blend with the IGHL or anterior capsule before inserting onto the base of the lesser tuberosity of the humerus. Variations of MGHL morphology produce variations in the size and position of the various synovial recesses of the shoulder.

Superior Glenohumeral Ligament

The superior glenohumeral ligament (SGHL) is found in 97% of shoulders and has a variety of origins.[28] The SGHL originates on the anterosuperior labrum, just anterior to the biceps anchor, with

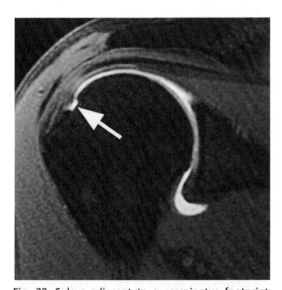

Fig. 22. Sulcus adjacent to supraspinatus footprint. Oblique coronal T1-weighted fat-suppressed image from an MR arthrogram demonstrates a small area of uncovered bone (*arrow*) interposed between the hyaline cartilage of the humeral head and the supraspinatus footprint. This should not be mistaken as a small partial undersurface tear.

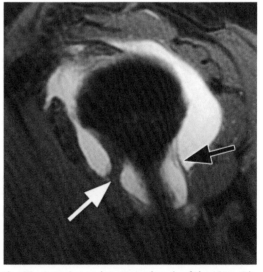

Fig. 23. Anterior and posterior bands of the IGHL. Oblique sagittal PD-weighted image from an MR arthrogram demonstrates the thick anterior band (*white arrow*) and thin posterior band (*black arrow*) of the IGHL.

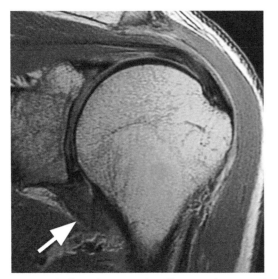

Fig. 24. Thickened IGHL and axillary pouch. Coronal oblique PD-weighted image of the shoulder demonstrates thickening of the IGHL and axillary pouch capsular fibers (*arrow*) in a patient with clinical findings of adhesive capsulitis.

a conjoined insertion with the MGHL or directly from the proximal biceps tendon (see **Fig. 18**).[24] A normal foramen is present between the SGHL and MGHL, which is responsible for the communication between the joint and the subscapularis bursa. It usually inserts superior to the lesser tuberosity, adjacent to the bicipital groove. The

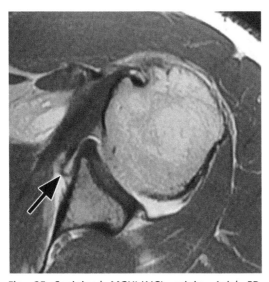

Fig. 25. Conjoined MGHL/AIGL origin. Axial PD-weighted image from an MR arthrogram shows the MGHL arising from the anterior scapular neck (*arrow*). More inferior images show this to be a conjoined origin with the AIGL (an anatomic variant).

SGHL is usually thin but may be thickened, particularly in cases where the MGHL is absent.

Capsular Variants

Three variants of the anterior and posterior joint capsule of the glenohumeral joint have been described. The capsule may insert on the glenoid margin (type I, 63% anterior/60% posterior), the glenoid neck (type II, 20% anterior/31% posterior), or more medially onto the scapula (type III, 17% anterior/9% posterior) (**Fig. 27**).[29,30] Types II and III seem to produce a capacious joint capsule that should not be mistaken for posttraumatic capsular laxity or capsular stripping. This can be falsely capacious when there is overdistention during MR arthrography or when the arm is overly internally or externally rotated. There is no correlation between redundancy of the anterior capsule and anterior instability.[3]

Labral Variants

The labrum is made of fibrous and fibrocartilagenous tissue that helps deepen the glenoid cavity. Variations of labral shape and configuration are common. As discussed previously, the labrum is a common insertion site for the long head of the biceps and the glenohumeral ligaments. The greatest morphologic variation of the labrum occurs at the 11-o'clock to 3-o'clock positions, near the insertion of many of the supporting capsular structures. These variations can be easily mistaken for labral or capsular pathology.

Also referred to as a sublabral hole, the sublabral foramen is an anatomic variation in the 1-o'clock to 3-o'clock positions of the anterosuperior labrum, where it is detached from the glenoid anteriorly and provides communication between the glenohumeral joint and the subscapular recess (**Fig. 28**). This is present in 8% to 18% of shoulders.[6] Although this is generally an incidental finding on MR arthrography, it may increase instability in patients with other lesions, in particular glenohumeral joint injury or a Bankart lesion.[6] On MR arthrography, it is an important variation to recognize because it can be misinterpreted as anterior extension of a SLAP tear. The medial margin of the detached labrum should appear smooth. If the medial free edge of the labrum appears irregular or intra-articular contrast extends between the labrum and glenoid to the 4-o'clock position, a SLAP tear should be suspected.[6] A sublabral foramen is frequently encountered on MR arthrography in association with a sublabral sulcus.

The sublabral sulcus or recess is defined as a gap between the biceps-labral complex and the superior glenoid with associated increased

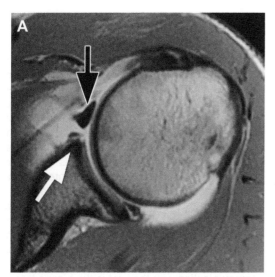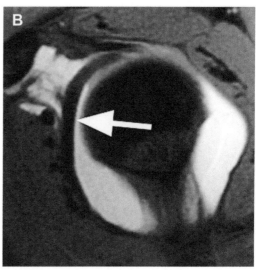

Fig. 26. Buford complex. Axial PD-weighted (*A*) and oblique sagittal T1-weighted (*B*) images from an MR arthrogram of the shoulder demonstrate an enlarged MGHL (*black arrow* in [*A*], *white arrow* in [*B*]) and a diminutive appearing anteroinferior labrum (*white arrow* in [*A*]).

mobility of the superior labrum. This occurs in type 2 and type 3 biceps-labral complexes where there is a predominant attachment of the biceps medial to the glenoid rim. This creates a potential space between the biceps-labral complex and the osseous glenoid that is easily seen on MR arthrography or when a large joint effusion is present. On diagnostic imaging or arthroscopy, the separation of the anterosuperior labrum from the glenoid can simulate a type II SLAP tear. Determination of

a normal sublabral sulcus is based on an equal width and depth and absence of the sulcus posterior to the insertion of the biceps on transverse images. On coronal images, the sulcus follows (is parallel to) the contour of the glenoid.[18] Signal abnormality extending perpendicular to this is diagnostic of a labral (SLAP) tear (**Fig. 29**). Intermediate signal intensity can be seen in the region of an expected sulcus or at other locations at the interface of the labrum and glenoid and is

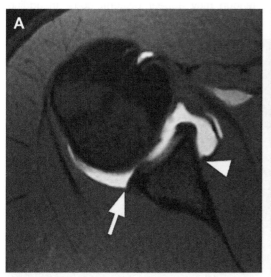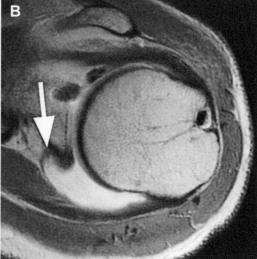

Fig. 27. Capsular insertions. (*A*) Axial T1-weighted fat-suppressed image from an MR arthrogram demonstrates a type 1 posterior capsular insertion (*arrow*) and a type 3 anterior capsular insertion (*arrowhead*). (*B*) Axial PD-weighted image from an MR arthrogram in a different patient demonstrates insertion of the posterior capsule more medially on the glenoid neck (*arrow*) consistent with a type 2 capsular insertion.

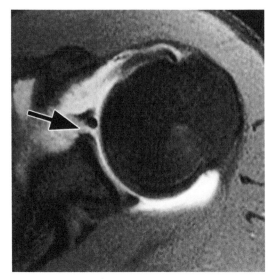

Fig. 28. Sublabral foramen. Axial T1-weighted image from an MR arthrogram demonstrates intra-articular gadolinium extending between the osseous glenoid and the anterosuperior labrum (*arrow*).

process. Because of this location, it can be confused for the subcoracoid bursa.[31] There is no communication between the glenohumeral joint and the subcoracoid bursa in healthy shoulders, although a communication between the sub-acromial-subdeltoid bursa and subcoracoid bursa may exist. The subscapular recess freely communicates with the glenohumeral joint via six possible synovial foramina located between the glenohumeral ligaments. The subscapular recess appears largest when the MGHL is absent or when the humerus is positioned in internal rotation, creating slack in the anterior capsule.[24] Positioning the shoulder in external rotation places tension on the subjacent subscapularis muscle and tendon, thereby compressing the recess, pushing joint fluid or arthrographic contrast into the glenohumeral joint.[6] Also in communication with the joint is the biceps tendon sheath, although in some postoperative patients, this communication is not seen possibly related to scarring or biceps tenodesis.

consistent with a transitional zone of histology between hyaline cartilage mixed with fibrous or fibrocartilaginous tissue (**Fig. 30**). This should also not be mistaken for a labral tear.[6]

JOINT RECESSES AND BURSAE

The subscapular recess is an extension of the glenohumeral joint, positioned posterior and anterosuperior to the subscapularis muscle and tendon, usually just underneath the coracoid

POSITIONAL VARIATIONS

The rotator cuff, in particular the supraspinatus and infraspinatus, is best imaged with a patient's shoulder placed in external rotation. When the humerus is internally rotated or overly externally rotated, the tendons are taken out of plane on standard oblique coronal and oblique sagittal imaging (**Fig. 31**). Increased overlap of the tendons occurs causing diagnostic uncertainty, particularly on oblique coronal images, where the supraspinatus tendon may appear discontinuous. In addition,

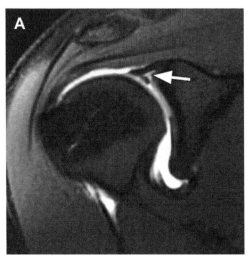
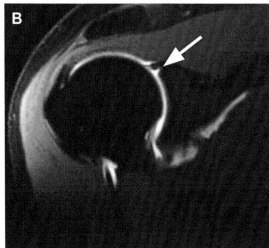

Fig. 29. SLAP tear and normal sublabral sulcus. (*A*) Coronal T1-weighted MR arthrographic images demonstrate bright signal abnormality extending into the substance of the superior labrum consistent with a SLAP tear (*arrow*) compared with the (*B*) normal sulcus seen in a different patient as bright signal paralleling the glenoid (*arrow*).

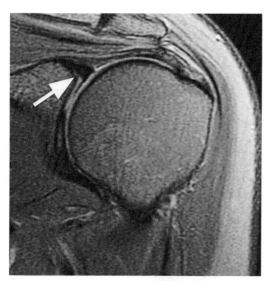

Fig. 30. Junctional zone of cartilage. Coronal PD-weighted fat-suppressed image demonstrates linear intermediate signal at the junction of the labrum and glenoid (*arrow*) consistent with a zone of transitional histology not to be mistaken for a labral tear.

imaging the rotator cuff in internal rotation bunches the anterior structures, creating artifactual signal abnormality and morphology of the subscapularis, MGHL, and capsular structures (**Fig. 32**). This

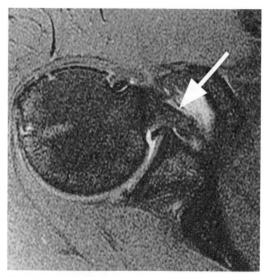

Fig. 32. Subscapularis bunching. Axial PD-weighted fat-suppressed image demonstrates an internally rotated shoulder with subsequent bunching of the subscapularis tendon creating artifactually increased intermediate signal (*arrow*) within the tendon that should not be mistaken for tendinosis.

positioning can also result in abnormal signal intensity between the supraspinatus and infraspinatus, likely due to magic angle artifact. Internal rotation makes imaging of the multipennate infraspinatus

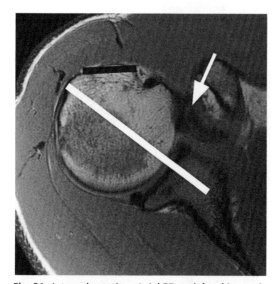

Fig. 31. Internal rotation. Axial PD-weighted image in a patient inappropriately positioned in internal rotation show bunching of the subscapularis tendon (*white arrow*). In addition, this position rotates the supraspinatus and its insertion (*black bar*) out of the plane that it is typically positioned in during external rotation (*white bar*). The oblique coronal plane is based on the expected orientation of the supraspinatus with external rotation.

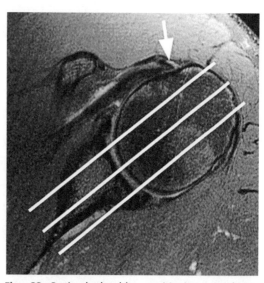

Fig. 33. Optimal shoulder positioning. Axial PD-weighted fat-suppressed image of the shoulder demonstrates a well-positioned, externally rotated shoulder with the bicipital groove present anterolaterally (*arrow*) and the course of the supraspinatus (*white lines*) perpendicular to the glenoid and parallel to the planned coronal plane of imaging.

tendon uniquely difficult. Because the infraspinatus tendon is rotated anteriorly, interposed muscle fibers between the tendons are visualized far laterally near the insertion of the cuff. External rotation of the shoulder positions the rotator cuff tendons parallel to the plane of section on coronal oblique images, allowing them to be seen throughout their length and, therefore, limiting diagnostic uncertainty (**Fig. 33**).[32]

Abduction and external rotation (ABER) of the shoulder is used to assess the glenohumeral ligaments and the anterior labrum in MR arthrography. ABER positioning of the shoulder works particularly well in assessing the structures of the anterior capsule, especially the anterior band of the glenohumeral ligament. The ABER position of the shoulder also accurately depicts the anterior capsule insertion site when imaging is comparable to gross dissection due to the tension placed on the anterior capsule. Thus, when MR arthrography is performed in cases where anterior instability is suspected, ABER imaging has been recommended to assess the anterior joint capsule, the anterior band of the IGHL, and anterior capsulolabral complex.[33] There remains some disagreement among radiologists, however, as to the necessity of ABER positioning in diagnosing the aforementioned labral and capsular pathology.

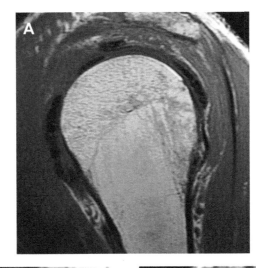

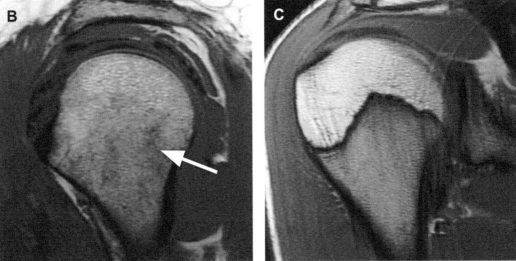

Fig. 34. Normal marrow signal. Oblique sagittal T1-weighted MR images in two adult patients show normal yellow marrow as diffuse and homogeneous bright signal (*A*) and normal hypointense red marrow (*B*) seen below the physeal scar (*white arrow*). Hypointense red marrow is normally seen in pediatric patients inferior to the pysis (*C*).

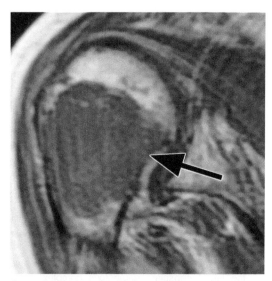

Fig. 35. Abnormal adult marrow. Coronal T1-weighted image demonstrates low-signal marrow throughout the humeral neck (*arrow*) in a patient with osseous metastatic disease from lung cancer.

BONE MARROW

Bone marrow heterogeneous signal is commonly seen within the humeral head and neck. Familiarity with the range of normal for different age groups is helpful to detect subtle marrow abnormalities as well as avoid unnecessary further imaging and possible intervention when variant, but benign, marrow signal is present. T1-weighted imaging is essential in evaluating bone marrow, because PD-weighted sequences can often mask significant intraosseous pathology. In adult patients, red marrow may be seen typically below the physeal scar as mildly hypointense signal on T1-weighted imaging (**Fig. 34**). With advanced anemia, red marrow conversion can become more pronounced spatially, extending down the humeral shaft and superiorly to subchondral bone. When the marrow signal becomes markedly low (hypointense to muscle), one must become concerned for a marrow infiltrative process, such as tumor (**Fig. 35**).

SUMMARY

The intricate anatomy of the shoulder is well delineated on MR imaging and MR arthrography. Accurate image interpretation requires knowledge of the diverse anatomic variants of the osseous, muscular, and capsulolabral structures of the shoulder. This knowledge is essential, because failure to recognize such variants can result in patients undergoing unnecessary therapy, including arthroscopy and attempted surgical repair.

REFERENCES

1. Bigliani LU, Ticker JB, Flatow EL, et al. The relationship of acromial architecture to rotator cuff disease. Clin Sports Med 1991;10(4):823–38.
2. Peh WCG, Farmer TH, Totty WG. Arcomial arch shape: assessment with MR imaging. Radiology 1995;195:501–5.
3. Stoller DW, Wolf EM, Li AE, et al. The shoulder. In: Stoller DW, Beltran S, Li AE, et al, editors. Magnetic resonance imaging in orthopedics and sports medicine, vol. 2. 3rd edition. Philadelphia: LWW; 2007. p. 1131–463.
4. Edelson TG, Taitz C. Anatomy of the coracoacromial arch. Relation to degeneration of the acromion. J Bone Joint Surg Br 1992;74(4): 589–94.
5. Gross A. [The incidence and role of os acromiale in the acromiohumeral impingement syndrome]. Radiol Med 1992;84:567–70 [in Italian].
6. Resnick D, Kang HS, Pretterklieber ML. Shoulder. In: Resnick D, Kang HS, Pretterklieber ML, editors. Internal derangements of the joints, vol. 1. 2nd edition. Philadelphia: Saunders Elsevier; 2007. p. 713–1122.
7. Park JG, Lee JK, Phelps CT. Os acromiale associated with rotator cuff impingement: MR imaging of the shoulder. Radiology 1994;193:255–7.
8. Richards RD, Sartoris DJ, Pathria MN, et al. Hill-Sachs lesion and normal humeral groove: MR imaging features allowing their differentiation. Radiology 1994;190:665–8.
9. Prescher A, Klumpen T. The glenoid notch and its relation to the shape of the glenoid cavity of scapula. J Anat 1997;190:457–60.
10. Inui H, Sugamoto K, Miyamoto T, et al. Evaluation of three dimensional glenoid structure using MRI. J Anat 2001;199:323–8.
11. Mulligan ME, Pontius CS. Posterior-inferior glenoid rim shapes by MR imaging. Surg Radiol Anat 2005;27:336–9.
12. Weishaupt D, Zanetti M, Nyffeler RW, et al. Posterior glenoid rim deficiency in recurrent (atraumatic) posterior shoulder instability. Skeletal Radiol 2000; 29:204–10.
13. Pal GP, Bhatt RH, Patel VS. Relationship between the tendon of the long head of the biceps brachii and the glenoid labrum in humans. Anat Rec 1991; 229:278–80.
14. Vangsness CT, Jorgenson SS, Watson T, et al. The origin of the long head of the biceps from the scapula and Glenoid Labrum. J Bone Joint Surg Br 1994;76:951–4.
15. Tuoheti Y, Itoi E, Minagawa H, et al. Attachment of the long head of the biceps tendon to the glenoid labrum and their relationships with the glenohumeral ligaments. Arthroscopy 2005;21(10):1242–9.

16. Yeh LR, Pedowitz R, Kwak S, et al. Intracapsular origin of the long head of the biceps tendon. Skeletal Radiol 1999;28:178–81.

17. MacDonald PB. Congenital anomaly of the biceps tendon and anatomy within the shoulder joint. Arthroscopy 1998;14:741–2.

18. Kwak SM, Brown RR, Resnick D, et al. Anatomy, anatomic variations and pathology of the 11- to 3-o'clock position of the glenoid labrum: findings on MR arthrography and anatomic sections. Am J Roentgenol 1998;171:235–8.

19. Hasehemi RH, Bradley WG Jr, Lisanti CJ. MRI the basics. 2nd edition. New York: LWW; 2004. p. 203–4.

20. Timins ME, Erickson SJ, Estowski LD, et al. Increased signal in the normal supraspinatus tendon on MR imaging: diagnostic pitfall caused by the magic angle effect. Am J Roentgenol 1995;164:109–14.

21. Erickson SJ, Cox IH, Hyde JS, et al. Effect of tendon orientation on MR imaging signal intensity: a manifestation of the "Magic Angle" phenomenon. Radiology 1991;181:389–92.

22. Ruotolo C, Fow JW, Nottage WM. The supraspinatus footprint: an anatomic study of the supraspinatus insertion. Arthroscopy 2004;20(3):246–9.

23. Minagawa H, Itoi E, Konno N. Humeral attachment of the supraspinatus and infraspinatus tendons: an anatomic study. Arthroscopy 1998;14(3):302–6.

24. Beltran J, Bencardino J, Mellado J, et al. MR arthrography of the shoulder: variants and pitfalls. Radiographics 1997;17:1403–12.

25. Beltran J, Bencardino J, Padron M, et al. The middle glenohumeral ligament: normal anatomy variants and pathology. Skeletal Radiol 2002;31:253–62.

26. Williams MM, Snyder SJ, Buford D. The Buford complex: a cordlike middle glenohumeral ligament and absent anterosuperior labrum complex—a normal anatomic capsulolabral variant. Arthroscopy 1994;10:241–7.

27. Tirman PF, Feller JF, Palmer WE, et al. The Buford complex—a variation of normal shoulder anatomy: MR arthrographic imaging features. Am J Roentgenol 1996;166:869–73.

28. Rockwood CA, Matsen FA. The shoulder. Philadelphia: Saunders; 1990. p. 17–27.

29. Zlatkin MB. Cross-sectional imaging of the capsular mechanism of the glenohumeral joint. Am J Roentgenol 1988;160:151.

30. Park YH, Lee JY, Moon SH, et al. MR arthrography of the labral capsular ligamentous complex in the shoulder: imaging variations and pitfalls. Am J Roentgenol 2000;175(3):667–72.

31. Schraner AB, Major NM. MR imaging of the subcoracoid bursa. Am J Roentgenol 1999;172(6):1567–71.

32. Davis SJ, Teresi LM, Bradley WG, et al. Effect of arm rotation on MR imaging of the rotator cuff. Radiology 1991;181:265–8.

33. Kwak SM, Brown RB, Trudell D, et al. Glenohumeral joint: comparison of shoulder positions at MR arthrography. Radiology 1998;208:375–80.

Elbow Magnetic Resonance Imaging Variants and Pitfalls

Marcos Loreto Sampaio, MD[a],*, Mark E. Schweitzer, MD[b]

KEYWORDS

- Elbow • MR imaging • Anatomy • Anatomic variation
- Pitfall • Ulnar nerve

Recognition of imaging variants has been appropriately stressed since not long after the first radiograph was performed. These variants are most disconcerting on more advanced imaging and in those parts of the body that are less imaged. Both of these qualifiers apply to magnetic resonance (MR) imaging of the elbow.

MR IMAGING FIELD INHOMOGENEITY

Inhomogeneities in the magnetic field and coil positioning can create areas of variable fat saturation or increased signal in tissues because of varying proximity to the coil, which may simulate bone marrow edema in the olecranon, bursitis in the adjacent subcutaneous tissues, or even tendinopathy in the tendinous insertions in the epicondyles.[1] As the elbow is often imaged away from the isocenter, inhomogeneous fat suppression is a particular problem. In the authors' experience, fat suppression creates the most diagnostic difficulties in the distal triceps and in the region of the olecranon bursa (**Fig. 1**).

The chemical shift artifact also creates difficulties in the interpretation of elbow MR imaging. The authors believe that these examinations of small parts are better done at 3 T, which presents with twice the chemical shift of 1.5 T. This artifact creates difficulties in interpreting cartilage defects presenting in the complex articular anatomy of the elbow.

The susceptibility artifact also creates a problem in the elbow related to the thick cortex of the distal humerus. This artifact, combined with chemical shift, may make subtle periosteal reaction and assessment of tumor spread more difficult.

BONE

Although bone marrow converts from distal to proximal, there are notable exceptions: larger areas of red marrow, which get left behind, and small islands of red marrow. With the increasing use of fat-suppressed imaging, these residual deposits create diagnostic dilemmas. In some patients, if not most patients, these red marrow islands can appear bright on fat-suppressed fluid-weighted or short time inversion recovery (STIR) images. The authors see this in several areas about the elbow, most commonly in the distal humeral metaphysis (**Fig. 2**) and the radial neck. It is the latter that can mimic a fracture, reactive changes to distal bicipital tendonitis, or even neoplasms.[2,3] The importance of these findings is multiple differential diagnosis, such as bone stress injuries, occult fractures, reactive marrow edema in epicondylitis, hydroxyapatite crystal deposition, osteochondral injuries, osteitis, osteomyelitis, and arthritis.[4–6] The clinical correlation and possible associated signal changes of the surrounding structures are important to determine in cases in which the marrow signal represents

---

The authors do not have any commercial relation to disclose.

[a] Musculoskeletal Radiology Department, The Ottawa Hospital, University of Ottawa, 501 Smyth Road, Module S, Ottawa, ON K1H 8L6, Canada

[b] Radiology Department, The Ottawa Hospital, University of Ottawa, 501 Smyth Road, Module S, Ottawa, ON K18 L6H, Canada

* Corresponding author.

E-mail address: msampaio@toh.on.ca

Magn Reson Imaging Clin N Am 18 (2010) 633–642
doi:10.1016/j.mric.2010.07.005

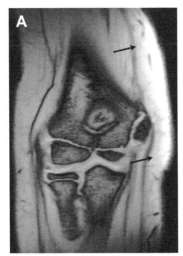

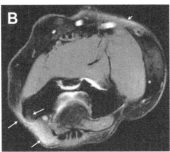

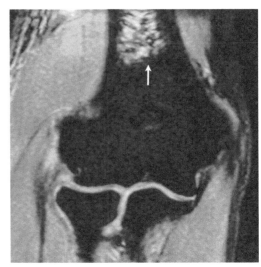

Fig. 2. Red marrow in the distal humerus. Coronal fluid-sensitive image with fat saturation. Residual red marrow in the distal humerus (*arrow*) is a common finding not to be mistaken for an abnormality.

Fig. 1. MR imaging field inhomogeneity. (*A*) Coronal gradient echo image. A large area of the subcutaneous tissue of the medial aspect of the distal arm (*arrows*) has higher intensity in relation to the adjacent areas because of the proximity to the coil. (*B*) Axial fluid-sensitive image with fat saturation. Insufficient fat saturation because of field inhomogeneity. The posteromedial subcutaneous fat and the periphery of the medial epicondyle (*arrows*) have an artifactual signal change that simulates edema. A similar, less prominent anterolateral artifactual abnormality (*small arrow*).

only a normal variant or a significant finding. Also, subchondral or subcortical predominance or marked signal increase in fluid-sensitive images favors a pathologic condition.

Another variation in the bone itself is activity-dependent cortical thickening of the humerus. This variation is not at all uncommon in even high-level recreational athletes such as tennis players and occurs as a response to the long-term upper limb activity.[7] For some reason, the humerus seems to disproportionately respond to stress. This should be differentiated from an overuse stress injury, although there really are different imaging appearances on the same spectrum. The more acute and potentially symptomatic bone responds with endosteal edema, often subtle

with periostitis. The latter is manifested by a thin line of bright T2 signal around the cortex.[5–7]

The supracondylar process of the humerus can be seen extending from the distal anteromedial humeral cortex and should not be mistaken for an osteochondroma. The supracondylar process is present in up to 2.7% of humans and is the origin of the ligament of Struthers, which extends distally on the medial epicondyle, forming an osteofibrous tunnel over the median nerve, and can be associated with compression neuropathy.[8] This is a well-known radiographic curiosity but may be disconcerting when seen on MR imaging for the first time.

In the ulna, a transverse trochlear ridge is seen along all the extension of the articular surface of the junction of the olecranon and coronoid process, which articulates with the humeral trochlea. It is 1 to 2 mm wide and usually has the same height, or it is just higher than the adjacent hyaline cartilage, and can be seen along the full transverse extension or partially in the radial or ulnar sides.[9] It was detected by Rosenberg and colleagues[9] in up to 81% of volunteers who underwent MR imaging of the elbow as a central elevation of the trochlear groove in sagittal images, in some cases with an irregular surface or even simulating an intraarticular osteophyte. The ulnar trochlear groove also has a waist in the junction between the olecranon and trochlea, where the ridge mentioned earlier is seen. This results in peripheral medial and lateral pseudodefects with cortical interruption in the articular surface, which should not be misinterpreted as an osteochondral lesion (**Fig. 3**).[9] That location, because it is a relative fossa, is one of the few places in the elbow proper that intraarticular bodies can deposit.

The pseudodefect of the capitellum is another anatomic variation frequently seen in the elbow. This is a result of the peculiar anatomy of the capitellum, which is wider anteriorly and superiorly, with almost twice the posterior width. In the posterior junction of the capitellum and the distal humerus, there is a groove and there are irregularities of the humeral surface extending laterally. This is identified in the MR imaging as a notch, deeper laterally, easily identified in sagittal images but also seen in the coronal plane. It can be more subtle or more conspicuous and can simulate an osteochondral lesion of the capitellum. Sometimes, a line with low signal can be seen extending proximally from the pseudodefect and should not be mistaken for a fracture (**Fig. 4**A).[9] The distinction between the pseudodefect and a true defect is based on anatomy. The variant is posterior. Osteochondral defects, Panner disease, and even geodes from arthritis tend to be anterior. The only exception to this rule is the impaction bruise, which occurs with transient subluxations and posterolateral rotatory instability. The bone bruise in this circumstance is also posterior (**Fig. 4**B).[10]

JOINT

Intraarticular inclusions are typical of synovial joints, such as the elbow. These can include fat pads, capsular rims (or synovial folds), menisci, and fibroadipose meniscoids.[11] The elbow has synovial folds or synovial plicae that are remnants of the embryologic formation of the joint.[12] The synovial folds have typical synovial membrane histology, with occasional polypoid projections, and low-signal intensity on MR imaging. The most frequent plicae is found in the posterosuperior olecranon recess, sometimes with a focal fat pad posterosuperiorly, but they can also be seen in the medial and lateral aspects of this recess or in the anterior humeral recess (**Fig. 5**A). These are usually asymptomatic, although repetitive injury may create an inflammatory reaction with thickening of the plica. Possible symptoms of a symptomatic plica include pain, joint locking, and snapping, simulating an intraarticular body, the so-called plica syndrome (**Fig. 5**B). Awaya and colleagues[12] studied cadavers and MR imaging of asymptomatic patients and found a posterosuperior plica in approximately 50% of asymptomatic patients, and in most cadavers, the plica measured approximately 1 or 2 mm, although in some cadavers, the plica measured 3 mm. In comparison, a symptomatic group was noted, in which the plicas tended to be thicker (3 mm) and had a histologic aspect of chronic synovitis. In the lateral aspect of the radiocapitellar joint, Huang and colleagues[13] also described a meniscus-like structure interposed between the capitellum and radial head, associated with painful snapping. In the same topography, Fukase and colleagues[14] described a thickened synovial fold with similar symptoms. The structures had a triangular or nodular aspect with low signal in the MR images and were identified respectively by an MR arthrogram and MR imaging, with a 47-mm surface coil for better resolution. Again, the observation of these structures should be correlated with clinical symptoms for proper diagnosis.

LIGAMENTS

The medial collateral ligament (or ulnar collateral ligament [UCL]) comprises 3 bundles: the anterior, the posterior, and the transverse. The anterior is the stronger, most important, and most frequently injured bundle, as it is the primary stabilizer of valgus stresses on the elbow. Clinically, the patient typically complains of pain in the acceleration phase of throwing.[15] The anterior bundle is well imaged in the coronal plane extending from the inferior surface of the medial epicondyle to insert on the periosteum of the medial aspect of the coronoid process of the ulna, in the sublime tubercle or up to 3 to 4 mm distal to it,[16] away from the articular margin. A thin lamina of fluid can be

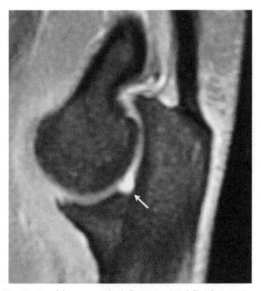

Fig. 3. Trochlear pseudodefect. Sagittal fluid-sensitive image with fat saturation, with a pseudodefect in the ulnar trochlea (*arrow*).

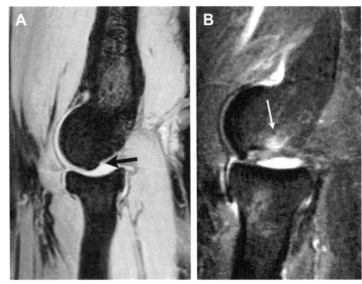

Fig. 4. Pseudodefect of the capitellum. Sagittal fluid-sensitive images with fat saturation. (*A*) The pseudodefect is localized posteriorly in the capitellum (*arrow*). (*B*) Impaction injury of the capitellum. The defect is irregular and there is marked marrow edema (*arrow*).

seen deep to the distal ligament insertion in this situation. Also, there is frequent fat interdigitation near its proximal insertion.[16] The normal ligament has low signal in both T1- and T2-weighted images, but fat signal can be seen in the proximal insertion as mentioned earlier, where the ligament is relatively wider (**Fig. 6**).[17] Because of this, Munshi and colleagues[16] recommend caution in the

diagnosis of partial tears of this ligament bundle considering the possible variable distance of its distal insertion. In pathologic cases, increased signal in T2-weighted images surrounding the ligament or ligament intrinsic signal change may be correlated to scar formation and rupture.[17]

The lateral collateral ligament (LCL) extends from the anteroinferior aspect of the lateral epicondyle to

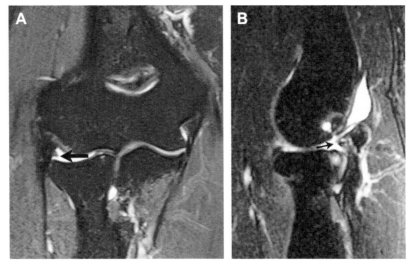

Fig. 5. Plica. (*A*) Coronal fluid-sensitive image with fat suppression. A lateral plica with meniscoid aspect (*arrow*) deep to the LCL. There were no clinical symptoms. (*B*) Sagittal fluid-sensitive, fat-suppressed image. Enlarged symptomatic posterolateral plica (*arrow*) with signal changes. There is also chondropathy of the radial head with bone marrow edema.

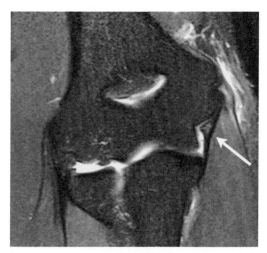

Fig. 6. UCL. Coronal fluid-sensitive image with fat suppression. The normal ligament has a proximal wider insertion (*arrow*). Fat in this topography can present with mild signal changes.

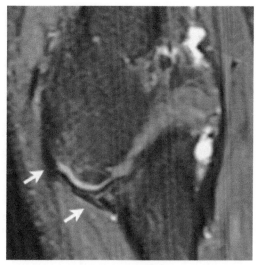

Fig. 7. Lateral collateral ulnar ligament. Coronal fluid-sensitive image with fat suppression. In this image, a normal lateral collateral ulnar ligament (*arrows*) is seen extending superolaterally from the supinator crest of the ulna toward the lateral epicondyle.

the radius. The LCL is also well seen on coronal images and has low signal on all pulse sequences. Adjacent to it, the previously described meniscus-like structure can be identified insinuating in the radiocapitellar joint (see **Fig. 5**A).

The lateral UCL extends posteriorly to the radial neck from the anteroinferior aspect of the lateral epicondyle to the supinator crest of the ulna. Together with the annular ligament and LCL, it is one of the most important lateral stabilizers of the elbow, and its acute or chronic disruption is related to the posterolateral rotatory instability.[18] Usually well observed in the coronal plane, this ligament is seen as a continuous low-signal structure (**Fig. 7**). The proximal origin, the most common location of tears, lies deep to the common extensor tendons and it can be indistinguishable from the origin of the LCL.[19] Also, partial volume averaging in the coronal plane, the magic angle effect, and ligament degeneration can create specious areas of high signal in the middle segment or contribute to poor visualization of the ligament.[18,19] The diagnosis of a tear should always take into account the clinical setting, image quality, imaging plane, and other associated image findings, such as positive pivot shift test, severe epicondylitis, previous history of surgery (particularly release of lateral tendons), posterior subluxation of the radial head in sagittal images, or even the patient's limitation to completely extend the elbow to do the MR imaging.[18–21]

TENDONS

The distal biceps brachii tendon is actually the coalescence of the tendons of the short and long

heads and inserts in the ulnar aspect of the bicipital tuberosity of the radius.[22] The bicipital tuberosity can have several different characteristics, and it was classified as smooth (or absent), small, medium, large single ridge (the most frequent type), and bifid (one medial and one lateral) by Mazzocca and colleagues[23] in a study of 178 cadavers with dissection and computed tomography. Erosion of the distal bicipital tendon by a prominent and irregular tuberosity during pronation was previously suggested,[23] although multiple factors are likely related to tendon disorders, such as intrinsic tendon degeneration, hypovascularity, spur in the bicipital tuberosity, and bicipitoradial bursitis.[22,23] Typically, the short-head tendon is proximally more medial and distally more anterior (**Fig. 8**). The short head inserts in the distal aspect of the tuberosity, although there are cases of distal tendon coalescence in which individual footprints are not well identified.[22]

The proximal aspect of the short-head distal tendon is also the origin of the lacertus fibrosus (the bicipital aponeurosis), which, if intact, can partially prevent the tendon's retraction (more than 8 cm of retraction are typically associated with a ruptured aponeurosis). This anatomic detail may help to differentiate a true partial of a coalesced tendon or a musculotendinous junction strain, usually treated conservatively, from a complete rupture of the individual distal tendon of one of the heads, which is more passive of surgical treatment.[24]

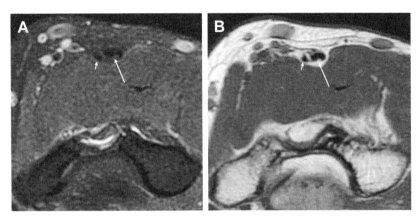

Fig. 8. Biceps brachii distal tendon. (*A*) Fluid-sensitive axial image with fat suppression and (*B*) T1-weighted axial image shows both short-head (*short arrow*) and long-head (*long arrow*) biceps tendons. This should not be mistaken for a tendon split.

At the triceps tendon insertion in the olecranon, a common distal tendon, comprising 3 tendon heads (lateral, long, and medial), can be seen, or a common tendon of only the long and lateral heads, more superficial, and seen separately from a deeper insertion of the medial head, which is mainly muscular. A possible explanation for that is the presence of fat infiltration within the distal fibers. This can mimic tendon degeneration or even interstitial tearing. The triceps is one of the visibly fasciculated tendons on MR imaging (as well as the quadriceps, rotator cuff, hamstrings, and Achilles). However, histologically, both are seen as a single insertion unit.[25] Sagittal images are usually more adequate for evaluation of this tendon (**Fig. 9**).

Cases of isolated partial or complete rupture of the medial head have been described, with integrity of the superficial tendon[25,26] and no palpable tendon gap. Clinically, these patients have a specific weakness to start the elbow extension when in full flexion. There are 2 reports of snapping elbow caused by the insinuation of the medial head peripherally to the medial epicondyle, which can be associated with ulnar neuropathy.[27] The medial head can also insert in the medial epicondyle or can simply be hypertrophic, resulting in compression of the ulnar nerve in the entrance of the cubital tunnel and neuropathy symptoms.[28]

BURSAE

The bicipitoradial bursa is localized between the smooth surface of the radial tuberosity and the biceps tendon reducing the local friction in pronation or supination. It can partially or completely envelop the distal tendon of the biceps close to its insertion and can therefore give the appearance of a synovial sheath.[29] However, the distal tendon

of the biceps brachii does not have a tendon sheath. The bursa can be identified with a thin volume of fluid within it (**Fig. 10**A). That should be differentiated from a pathologic bursa as

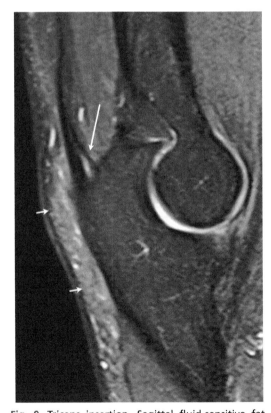

Fig. 9. Triceps insertion. Sagittal fluid-sensitive fat-suppressed image. A small area of high signal intensity within the tendon insertion (*long arrow*) is a possible normal finding. In this same image, the small arrows indicate mild edema in the olecranon subcutaneous tissues, a frequent nonsymptomatic finding.

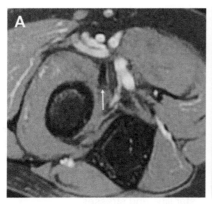
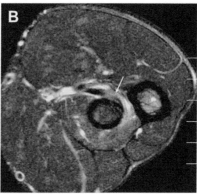

Fig. 10. Bicipitoradial bursa. Axial fluid-sensitive fat-suppressed images. (*A*) The subtle high-signal intensity surrounding the distal biceps brachii tendon (*arrow*) represents a normal bursa. (*B*) Partial tear of the biceps tendon (*arrow*), with increased intrinsic signal intensity and fluid in the adjacent bicipitoradial bursa (bursitis).

a result of repetitive mechanical trauma (most frequently) because of increased forearm rotation or infection, inflammatory arthropathy, chemical synovitis, bone proliferation or bicipital tuberosity irregularities, and synovial chondromatosis.[29] Some investigators believe that this is an anatomic bursa seen in all patients. However, if it is visible, in the authors' opinion, it should be considered abnormal (**Fig. 10B**).

The olecranon bursa provides smooth movement between the skin and the olecranon.[30] Repetitive minor traumas to the bursa (student's elbow) can result in a nonspecific bursitis or simply subcutaneous thickening or callus formation. Also, obesity, septic or inflammatory arthropathy such as gout and rheumatoid arthritis, and even a triceps tendon rupture can be underlying causes of bursitis. *Staphylococcus aureus* is the most frequent agent involved in septic bursitis, more frequently seen in patients who are alcohol abusers; patients who use steroids; or those who have diabetes, renal impairment, or malignancy.[30] Also, mild MR signal changes in the subcutaneous tissues adjacent to the olecranon with clear definition of a bursa may be seen representing a callus (**Figs. 9 and 11**). The authors believe any visible fluid here is also a sign of bursitis. However, many patients develop skin thickening over the olecranon process. This can obscure the normal subcutaneous fat that is used as a sign to exclude bursitis. As discussed earlier, this is an area that is rife with inhomogeneous fat suppression, which can cause the specious appearance of bursitis.

NEUROVASCULAR

The ulnar nerve travels along the posteromedial aspect of the distal arm medially to the triceps muscle and then enters the cubital tunnel,

emerging distally between the 2 heads of the flexor carpi ulnaris and then between that and the flexor digitorum profundus.[31]

The cubital tunnel, the fibro-osseous tunnel containing the ulnar nerve, is delimited by the olecranon laterally, medial epicondyle medially, the transverse and posterior bundle of the UCL and the capsule (floor), and superficially by the aponeurosis of the flexor carpi ulnaris distally and proximally by the retinaculum (often called the Osborne band), with perpendicular fibers in relation to the aponeurosis.[32]

Anatomic variations of the cubital tunnel have been described. O'Driscoll and colleagues[32] divided the cubital tunnel into 4 categories: type 0 with absent retinaculum and dislocated ulnar

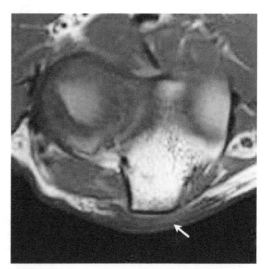

Fig. 11. Callus. Axial T1-weighted image. The arrow indicates signal change in the subcutaneous tissues superficial to the olecranon.

nerve, type Ia with normal retinaculum, taut in flexion but without compression of the nerve, type Ib with a pathologically thick retinaculum chronically compressing the nerve, and type 2 with an anconeus epitrochlearis muscle substituting the retinaculum. This muscle is probably atavistic in humans, sometimes considered an accessory to the medial head of the triceps, and is present in 3% to 28% of cadaver elbows (**Fig. 12**).[32] Even though considered a variant, this accessory muscle, like those seen in the tarsal tunnel of the foot, may cause symptoms, in this case ulnar neuritis.

Medial subluxation or even dislocation of the ulnar nerve over the tip of the medial epicondyle can be observed, even without the presence of clinical symptoms, although this may increase the probability of nerve injuries. Usually that happens with the flexion of the elbow (approximately 16% of the population[32]), but in some cases, the ulnar nerve may be subluxated or dislocated even in an extended elbow. To some degree, the variation of a hypoplastic groove is the cause of this subluxation. Therefore, the subluxability of the ulnar nerve is a result of an interaction between anatomy (groove shape), dynamic stability, and stresses.

The ulnar nerve is usually round or oval in the cubital tunnel,[31] has a constant cross-sectional area across the elbow (**Fig. 13**), and is usually isointense in relation to the muscles.[33] In elbow flexion, the pressure of the cubital tunnel increases, and the nerve becomes flat. If you happen to image in this position, beware of this variant, because it is not always a sign of cubital tunnel syndrome.

The nerve can also have a high signal in fluid-weighted images, for example as a consequence of the magic angle phenomenon; sometimes it is

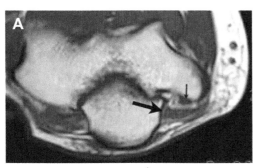

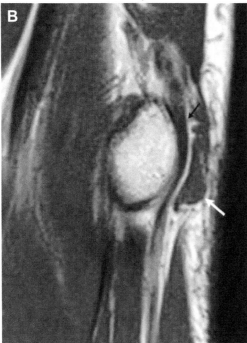

Fig. 12. Anconeus epitrochlearis. Axial (*A*) and sagittal (*B*) T1-weighted images show an accessory muscle (anconeus epitrochlearis) (*large arrow*) overlying the ulnar nerve (*small arrow*). In this case, there were no symptoms of ulnar neuritis. The ulnar nerve has typical width along the cubital tunnel. Note the thin normal surrounding fat.

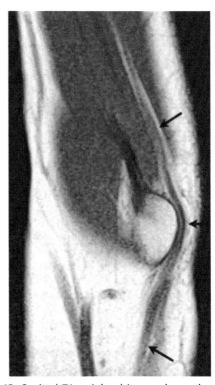

Fig. 13. Sagittal T1-weighted image shows the ulnar nerve (*arrows*) with constant diameter along the distal humerus and proximal forearm. Note the normal surrounding fat plane. The middle arrow indicates the cubital tunnel segment.

at approximately 55° in relation to the B0 magnetic field because of obliquity and the patient's positioning. When we see high signal within the nerve, we assess how long the segment of abnormal signal is. The longer it is, the more likely it is a variant. Our general rule is pathology should be 4 axial images or less.

In addition, minor enlargement of the nerve is not specific for a pathologic condition. Britz and colleagues[33] correlated MR imaging, electrodiagnostic evaluation, and clinical intraoperative findings, and found that in patients with ulnar neuropathy, both increased signal and enlargement of the nerve were usually found above and below the distal humerus between 27 mm and 4 mm and between 19 mm and 8 mm, respectively (**Fig. 14**).

SOFT TISSUES

There are 2 common sites where lymph nodes can simulate masses on routine joint MR imaging, the popliteal node posterior to the femur, and the medial epitrochlear lymph node adjacent to the elbow. This node may show high-signal intensity in fluid-weighted images. Although this node is a normal structure, the authors believe that if it is more than subtly seen, it is pathologic. This node can be involved in association with rheumatoid arthritis, systemic lupus erythematous, cat-

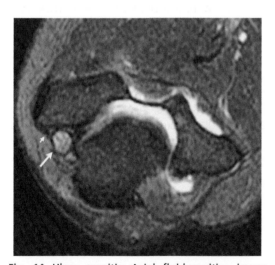

Fig. 14. Ulnar neuritis. Axial fluid-sensitive image with fat saturation. An enlarged ulnar nerve (*large arrow*) with increased signal intensity is seen in the cubital tunnel. The cubital tunnel retinaculum insertion in the medial epicondyle (*small arrow*). In some patients, variations of the retinaculum may result in nerve subluxation or dislocation and ulnar neuropathy. In this case, the retinaculum has a typical appearance.

scratch disease, tuberculosis, lymphoproliferative disorders, and rarely because of metastatic involvement.[34,35] Tumoral lymph nodes tend to be rounded and better defined, with less adjacent soft tissue stranding and edema than infectious lymph nodes, which are enlarged and associated with adjacent soft tissue edema and stranding and heterogeneous gadolinium enhancement.[34]

REFERENCES

1. Kijowski R, De Smet AA. Magnetic resonance imaging findings in patients with medial epicondylitis. Skeletal Radiol 2005;34(4):196–202.
2. Richardson ML, Patten RM. Age-related changes in marrow distribution in the shoulder: MR imaging findings. Radiology 1994;192(1):209–15.
3. Berg BCV, Malghem J, Lecouvet FE, et al. Magnetic resonance imaging of the normal bone marrow. Skeletal Radiol 1998;27(9):471–83.
4. Bui-Mansfield LT, Moak M. Magnetic resonance appearance of bone marrow edema associated with hydroxyapatite deposition disease without cortical erosion. J Comput Assist Tomogr 2005; 29(1):103–7.
5. Lee JC, Malara FA, Wood T, et al. MRI of stress reaction of the distal humerus in elite tennis players. AJR Am J Roentgenol 2006;187(4):901–4.
6. Hoy G, Wood T, Phillips N, et al. When physiology becomes pathology: the role of magnetic resonance imaging in evaluating bone marrow oedema in the humerus in elite tennis players with an upper limb pain syndrome. Br J Sports Med 2006;40(8):710–3 [discussion: 713].
7. Haapasalo H, Kontulainen S, Sievänen H, et al. Exercise-induced bone gain is due to enlargement in bone size without a change in volumetric bone density: a peripheral quantitative computed tomography study of the upper arms of male tennis players. Bone 2000;27(3):351–7.
8. Pećina M, Borić I, Anticević D. Intraoperatively proven anomalous Struthers' ligament diagnosed by MRI. Skeletal Radiol 2002;31(9):532–5.
9. Rosenberg ZS, Beltran J, Cheung YY. Pseudodefect of the capitellum: potential MR imaging pitfall. Radiology 1994;191(3):821–3.
10. Rosenberg ZS, Blutreich SI, Schweitzer ME, et al. MRI features of posterior capitellar impaction injuries. Am J Roentgenol 2008;190:435–41.
11. Mercer SR, Bogduk N. Intra-articular inclusions of the elbow joint complex. Clin Anat 2007;20(6): 668–76.
12. Awaya H, Schweitzer ME, Feng A, et al. Elbow synovial fold syndrome: MR imaging findings. Am J Roentgenol 2001;177:1377–81.
13. Huang GS, Lee CH, Lee HS, et al. A meniscus causing painful snapping of the elbow joint: MR

imaging with arthroscopic and histologic correlation. Eur Radiol 2005;15(12):2411–4.

14. Fukase N, Kokubu T, Fujioka H, et al. Usefulness of MRI for diagnosis of painful snapping elbow. Skeletal Radiol 2006;35(10):797–800.

15. Rahman RK, Levine WN, Ahmad CS. Elbow medial collateral ligament injuries. Curr Rev Musculoskelet Med 2008;1(3–4):197–204.

16. Munshi M, Pretterklieber ML, Chung CB, et al. Anterior bundle of ulnar collateral ligament: evaluation of anatomic relationships by using MR imaging, MR arthrography, and gross anatomic and histologic analysis. Radiology 2004;231(3):797–803.

17. Nakanishi K, Masatomi T, Takahiro O, et al. MR arthrography of elbow: evaluation of the ulnar collateral ligament of elbow. Skeletal Radiol 1996;25(7):629–34.

18. Terada N, Yamada H, Toyama YJ. The appearance of the lateral ulnar collateral ligament on magnetic resonance imaging. J Shoulder Elbow Surg 2004; 13(2):214–6.

19. Carrino JA, Morrison WB, Zou KH, et al. Lateral ulnar collateral ligament of the elbow: optimization of evaluation with two-dimensional MR imaging. Radiology 2001;218(1):118–25.

20. Bredella MA, Tirman PF, Fritz RC, et al. MR imaging findings of lateral ulnar collateral ligament abnormalities in patients with lateral epicondylitis. AJR Am J Roentgenol 1999;173(5):1379–82.

21. Sanal HT, Chen L, Haghighi P, et al. Annular ligament of the elbow: MR arthrography appearance with anatomic and histologic correlation. AJR Am J Roentgenol 2009;193(2):W122–6.

22. Athwal GS, Steinmann SP, Rispoli DM. The distal biceps tendon: footprint and relevant clinical anatomy. J Hand Surg Am 2007;32(8):1225–9.

23. Mazzocca AD, Cohen M, Berkson E, et al. The anatomy of the bicipital tuberosity and distal biceps tendon. J Shoulder Elbow Surg 2007;16(1):123.

24. Koulouris G, Malone W, Omar IM, et al. Bifid insertion of the distal biceps brachii tendon with isolated rupture: magnetic resonance findings. J Shoulder Elbow Surg 2009;18(6):e22–5.

25. Belentani C, Pastore D, Wangwinyuvirat M, et al. Triceps brachii tendon: anatomic-MR imaging study in cadavers with histologic correlation. Skeletal Radiol 2009;38(2):171–5.

26. Athwal GS, McGill RJ, Rispoli DM. Isolated avulsion of the medial head of the triceps tendon: an anatomic study and arthroscopic repair in 2 cases. Arthroscopy 2009;25(9):983–8.

27. Dreyfuss U, Kessler I. Snapping elbow due to dislocation of the medial head of the triceps. A report of two cases. J Bone Joint Surg Br 1978;60(1):56–7.

28. Boero S, Sénès FM, Catena N. Pediatric cubital tunnel syndrome by anconeus epitrochlearis: a case report. J Shoulder Elbow Surg 2009;18 (2):e21–3.

29. Skaf AY, Boutin RD, Dantas RW, et al. Bicipitoradial bursitis: MR imaging findings in eight patients and anatomic data from contrast material opacification of Bursae followed by routine radiography and MR imaging in cadavers. Radiology 1999;212:111–6.

30. Floemer F, Morrison WB, Bongartz G, et al. MRI characteristics of olecranon bursitis. Am J Roentgenol 2004;183:29–34.

31. Kim YS, Yeh LR, Trudell D, et al. MR imaging of the major nerves about the elbow: cadaveric study examining the effect of flexion and extension of the elbow and pronation and supination of the forearm. Skeletal Radiol 1998;27(8):419–26.

32. O'Driscoll SW, Horii E, Carmichael SW. The cubital tunnel and ulnar neuropathy. J Bone Joint Surg Br 1991;73(4):613–7.

33. Britz GW, Haynor DR, Kuntz C, et al. Ulnar nerve entrapment at the elbow: correlation of magnetic resonance imaging, clinical, electrodiagnostic, and intraoperative findings. Neurosurgery 1996;38(3): 458–65 [discussion: 465].

34. Gielen J, Wang XL, Vanhoenacker F, et al. Lymphadenopathy at the medial epitrochlear region in cat-scratch disease. Eur Radiol 2003;13(6):1363–9.

35. Selby CD, Marcus HS, Toghill PJ. Enlarged epitrochlear lymph nodes: an old physical sign revisited. J R Coll Physicians Lond 1992;26(2):159–61.

Pitfalls of Wrist MR Imaging

W. James Malone, DO[a],*, Robert Snowden, MD[a], Fozail Alvi, MD[a], Joel C. Klena, MD[b]

KEYWORDS

- Triangular fibrocartilage • Wrist ligaments • Carpal boss
- Ulnar abutment • Lunate avascular necrosis
- Magnetic resonance imaging

WRIST IMAGING

The multiplanar capability coupled with excellent tissue contrast makes magnetic resonance (MR) imaging the ideal imaging modality to evaluate for myotendinous, ligamentous, and bone pathology in any joint. MR imaging of the hand and wrist has lagged behind that for other joints, in part because of the difficulty in accurately evaluating the diminutive anatomic structures. Technology such as improved coils, 3-T imaging, and short-bore open systems built to comfortably image the upper extremity have proved to increase the utility of MR imaging of the wrist. This article reviews fundamental pearls and pitfalls with corresponding images from 1.5-T systems that the practicing radiologist must be mindful of to provide clinically relevant information to the ordering doctor.

WRIST ALIGNMENT

The normal anatomic relationships of the carpus have been validated over decades with standardized reproducible positioning for posteroanterior (PA) and lateral radiographs. For example, the standard radiographic PA view of the wrist is obtained with the wrist flat on the x-ray table, the shoulder abducted 90°, and the elbow flexed 90°.[1] Once obtained, there are criteria that the radiologist can use to verify the images are satisfactory, which on the lateral view is based on the location of the extensor carpi ulnaris groove and

on the PA radiograph is based on the location of the pisiform with respect to the palmar surface of the capitate and scaphoid.[2–4] These anatomic relationships are important because poorly positioned radiographs may simulate pathology, such as carpal instability.

By contrast, positioning for MR imaging is variable. The wrist may be imaged at one's side for those few patients who fit the bore of the magnet in this position. This position is comfortable, but the wrist is out of the isocenter of the magnet, which in turn decreases signal to noise and makes fat suppression more difficult. Alternatively, the superman position (prone position with arm extended) is commonly used for those who are able to tolerate the position. The benefit here is that the wrist is more in the center of the magnet bore, but the position is less comfortable for elderly patients and those with breathing difficulties. Regardless of position, the degree of pronation and supination, ulnar and radial deviation, and grip varies somewhat from patient to patient. As with poorly positioned radiographs, there is the possibility of misinterpreting pathology due to wrist positioning rather than a true pathologic process.

Static carpal instability may be diagnosed with radiographs based on classic anatomic relationships.[5] Two examples of this are volar intercalated segmental instability (VISI) and dorsal intercalated segmental instability (DISI). Patients with DISI demonstrate dorsal tilting of the lunate and those

[a] Department of Radiology, MC 20-07, Geisinger Medical Center, 100 North Academy Avenue, Danville, PA 17822, USA
[b] Department of Orthopedic Surgery, Geisinger Medical Center, 100 North Academy Avenue, Danville, PA 17822, USA
* Corresponding author.
E-mail address: wjmalone@geisinger.edu

with VISI demonstrate volar tilting of the lunate. The diagnosis is confirmed by measuring the scapholunate (SL) and capitolunate (CL) angles obtained from the true lateral radiograph (**Fig. 1**).

DISI is diagnosed with a CL angle greater than SL angle of more than 80°. An SL greater than 60° but less than 80° is suspicious for DISI. VISI is diagnosed by demonstrating a CL angle less than −30° and SL angle less than 30°.[6,7]

A "pseudo DISI configuration" is commonly seen on sagittal MR images, particularly when imaging in the "superman" position (**Fig. 2**). This image may be the result of different mechanical load on the wrist in this position compared with that of the lateral radiograph.[7] To avoid this pitfall, radiographic correlation is recommended before making the diagnosis of DISI or VISI on MR imaging. This correlation is particularly important in the absence of an SL and lunotriquetral (LT) ligament tear, which would support the diagnosis of DISI and VISI, respectively.

On standard PA radiographs, the articular surfaces of the ulna and radius are at the same level, termed neutral ulnar variance. With negative ulnar variance the radius projects more distal to the ulna, and with positive ulnar variance the radius projects proximal to the ulna (**Fig. 3**).[8,9] However, it is important to consider that wrist position and grip are significant determinants of ulnar variance. For example, ulnar positive variance increases with pronation and increased grip, and vice versa[10–12] Thus, given the variability of wrist positioning on MR imaging, subtle isolated ulnar variance should not be diagnosed without first correlating with radiographs.[8] Furthermore, in the presence of classic findings, the apparent lack of ulnar variance should not deter one from diagnosing ulnar impaction in the absence of ulnar positive variance, or Kienbock disease in the absence of negative ulnar variance.

WRIST BONE

Ulnar impaction syndrome (also known as ulnar abutment) is secondary to abnormal loading of the wrist, resulting in progressive pain from

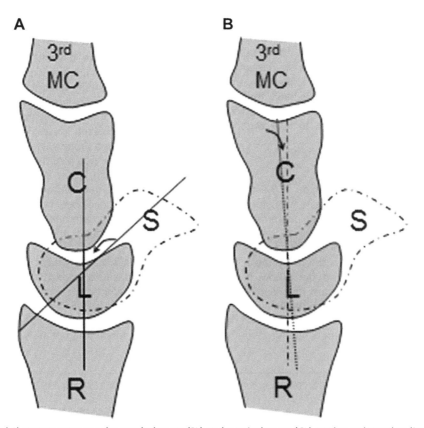

Fig. 1. (*A* and *B*) How to measure the scapholunate (SL) and captitolunate (CL) angles on lateral radiographs. In *A*, a line is drawn through the axis of the scaphoid (S) and then the lunate (L). The SL angle is denoted by the curved arrow. Normal is 30° to 60°. In *B*, lines are drawn through the axis of the lunate (L) and the capitate (C). Curved arrow denotes the CL angle. Normal angle is −30° to 30°. 3rd MC, third metacarpal base; R, radius.

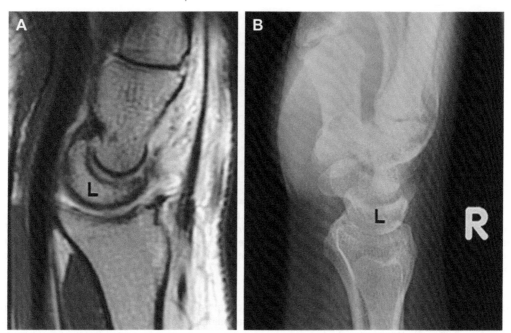

Fig. 2. (*A*) Dorsal tilting of the lunate (L) on MR imaging, suspicious for DISI. No accompanying ligamentous injury was present on MR imaging. (*B*) True lateral radiograph in the same patient demonstrating no dorsal tilting, and therefore the apparent DISI on MR imaging was actually false positive due to positioning.

impaction of the ulnar head against the lunate and triquetrum across a thinned or torn triangular fibrocartilage (TFC).[13] Ulnar positive variance is classically present, but not always.[14] The constellation of MR imaging findings seen with ulnar impaction include: central TFC thinning or tear, progressive cartilage loss, signal alteration in the ulnar head and adjacent ulnar aspect of the lunate and/or triquetrum, and LT ligament tear (**Figs. 4** and **5**).[15,16] These findings typically follow the aforementioned progression, closely reflecting Palmer's classification system of degenerative TFC tears.[17,18] Depending on the stage of the disease, the bony signal alteration may be that of fluid (low T1 and high T2 signal) or sclerosis (low T1 and low T2

signal).[17] It is important that findings suggesting ulnar impaction syndrome be noted, in addition to diagnosing the central TFC tear, as treatment is not simple arthroscopic debridement as with symptomatic central TFC tear. The accompanying force imbalance at the ulnar head must be addressed (ulnar positive variance), which often requires resection of the distal ulna.[19]

Additional conditions, such as Kienbock disease and carpal cysts, may mimic ulnar impaction on MR imaging. Incidental carpal cysts are frequent throughout the carpus. These cysts often form along ligamentous attachments, and therefore centrally located carpal bones like the lunate and capitate are frequently affected. The cysts may

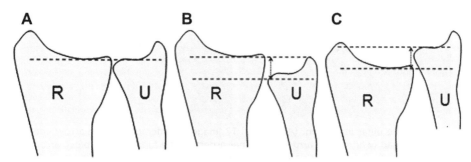

Fig. 3. (*A–C*) Neutral, negative, and positive ulnar variance, respectively. R, radius; U, ulna.

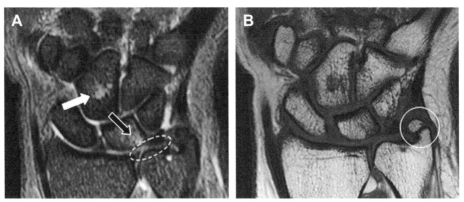

Fig. 4. (A and B) Classic but relatively mild ulnar impaction. (A) A coronal T2 image demonstrating a full-thickness tear of triangular fibrocartilage complex (TFC) (*dashed circle*) with marrow edema at the ulnar aspect of the lunate (*black arrow*). Note incidental capitate cyst (*white arrow*). (B) Coronal T1 image of the same patient demonstrating incidental nonunion of ulnar styloid (*white circle*), which was not well visualized on coronal T2 image.

appear as small peripheral erosions at the ligament attachment, or may tunnel into the center of the bone (**Fig. 6**). When signal changes are present in the lunate, distinction must be made between ulnar impaction syndrome, lunate cysts (**Fig. 7**), and Kienbock disease. Both conditions are distinguished from ulnar impaction based on the location of the signal alteration in the lunate, which in ulnar impaction is limited to its ulnar side.[9,16,17] Furthermore, with Kienbock disease the signal changes are typically more confluent (**Fig. 8**), and may be accompanied by lunate collapse (**Fig. 9**).

Distinction must be made between ulnar impaction and other similarly termed but separate syndromes that are also known to cause ulnar-sided wrist pain.[17] Ulnar impingement is a condition whereby a short distal ulna impinges on the distal radius at the sigmoid notch, resulting in a painful and disabling pseudoarthrosis.[20] Ulnar styloid impaction is similar, but the bony impaction is between the ulnar styloid and triquetrum, which is thought to be caused by morphologic changes in the ulnar styloid or nonunion of prior ulnar styloid fracture.[17]

Large carpal cysts were demonstrated previously, but they vary in size and may be isolated or numerous (**Fig. 10**). On MR imaging, both nutrient vessels and carpal cysts have been shown to mimic the early erosions of rheumatoid arthritis (RA), which may all develop in similar locations and commonly are present along ligament attachments.[21,22] The distinction is not difficult in the later stages of RA, because the erosions are by then numerous and characteristic in location (**Fig. 11**). However, it is preferable to make the

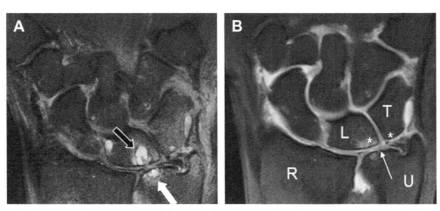

Fig. 5. (A and B) Severe ulnar impaction. (A) Coronal T2 image that demonstrates marrow edema and cystic change in the ulnar head (*white block arrow*) and ulnar aspect of the lunate (*black block arrow*). (B) Coronal T1 arthrographic sequence showing associated full-thickness central TFC tear (*white line arrow*). Note absence of LT ligament (*between asterisks*). L, lunate; R, radius; T, triquetrum; U, ulna.

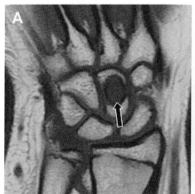
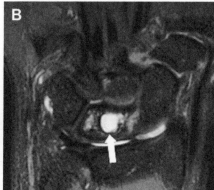

Fig. 6. (*A* and *B*) Two different patients with incidental carpal cysts. (*A*) T1 image showing a large central capitate cyst (*black arrow*). (*B*) T2 image demonstrating a large central lunate cyst (*white arrow*).

diagnosis of RA early in the disease process to implement treatment as early as possible to prevent joint destruction. In this situation, scrutinizing the MR images for associated findings typical of RA, for example, synovitis and tenosynovitis (**Fig. 12**), as well as correlating the clinical signs and symptoms and serologic workup, are all recommended.[23]

CARPAL BOSS

The carpal boss is a bony excrescence off the dorsal wrist, which is a long known, but often overlooked cause of wrist pain (**Fig. 13**). Although the etiology remains unclear, some have reported a posttraumatic cause of the deformity.[24] Others believe it is a developmental anomaly known as the os styloidium; an accessory ossification center that is located in the area of the quadrangular trapezoid-capitate-metacarpal joint.[25] The carpal boss varies in size and may be either completely

isolated, or more commonly it is fused to the dorsal aspect of the second or third metacarpal, or occasionally to the capitate or trapezoid.[26] Many patients with carpal bossing are asymptomatic. Symptomatic carpal boss (**Fig. 14**) typically presents in the fourth decade with the dominant hand being more commonly affected.[25,27] The altered biomechanics may result in overlying extensor tendinopathy, ganglion formation or bursitis, and eventually arthrosis.[25,26] Treatment is surgical for those who fail conservative management, with wide excision of the carpal boss balanced with the risk of developing subsequent joint instability.[28,29]

TYPE II LUNATE

The presence of a medial lunate facet that articulates with the hamate has been termed a type II lunate (**Fig. 15**).[30] The type II lunate configuration has a reported incidence of 44% to 77% and is

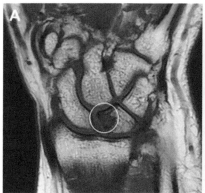
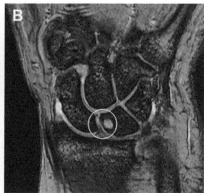
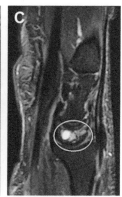

Fig. 7. (*A–C*) A lunate cyst, which could mimic ulnar impaction. (*A* and *B*) Coronal T1- and T2-weighted images, respectively, in the same patient, demonstrating a lunate cyst (*circle*). (*C*) Corresponding sagittal T2 image demonstrating the same incidental lunate cyst (*oval*). This condition can be distinguished from ulnar impaction because of its location away from the ulnar aspect of the lunate. This cyst was thought to be the sequela of prior trauma.

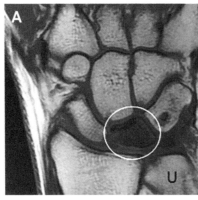
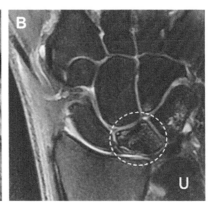

Fig. 8. (*A* and *B*) Classic Kienbock disease. (*A*) Coronal T1 image demonstrating diffuse loss of T1 marrow signal in the lunate (*circle*). (*B*) Corresponding coronal T2 image demonstrating mild patchy edema in the lunate (*dashed circle*).

associated with an increased incidence of chondromalacia in the proximal pole of the hamate.[30–34] The size of this extra-articular facet ranges from 1 mm to up to 12 mm, with most in the 2- to 4.5-mm range.[34]

The majority of wrists with a type II facet demonstrate no corresponding abnormality; however, cartilage loss, marrow edema, and subchondral cystic change on MR imaging indicate developing arthrosis (**Fig. 16**). It has been shown that the incidence of proximal hamate chondromalacia at arthroscopy and gross dissection is greater than that reported by MR imaging alone, indicating that many cases are occult on MR imaging.[30,31,34] This discrepancy may be caused by the relatively thin hyaline articular cartilage layers of the radiocarpal and intercarpal joints, resulting in difficulties in their visualization.[35,36] When present, marrow edema in the proximal hamate is nonspecific and can be similar to that seen in patients with carpal contusion or fractures.[34] However, in the presence

of a type II lunate, chondromalacia should be strongly considered, particularly in the absence of trauma and when the edema is at the articulation of the hamate and lunate. Surgery has been shown to be beneficial in some patients with chronic wrist pain due to hamatolunate arthrosis. In 2 series of patients, resolution of symptoms was achieved following surgical resection of the diseased proximal pole of the hamate.[37,38]

WRIST TENDONS

On wrist MR imaging, tendinopathy is denoted by intrasubstance signal alteration within a flexor or extensor tendon. However, asymptomatic or falsely increased intrasubstance signal alteration can be seen in the flexor and extensor tendons of the wrist, and therefore one must be mindful of this potential pitfall.[39] Commonly implicated in this finding is the phenomenon known as magic angle. Magic angle is rampant in musculoskeletal

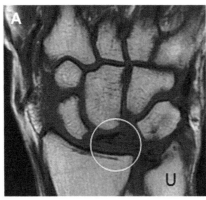
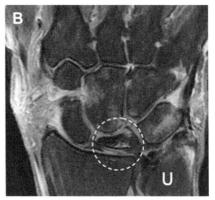

Fig. 9. (*A* and *B*) Kienbock disease with lunate collapse. (*A*) Coronal T1 image demonstrating diffuse loss of T1 marrow signal in the lunate with associated flattening (*circle*). (*B*) Corresponding coronal T2 image demonstrating areas of mild patchy edema in the collapsed lunate (*dashed circle*). U, ulna.

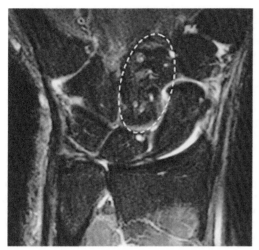

Fig. 10. Coronal T2 sequences in a patient with numerous tiny cysts throughout the carpal bones, greatest in the capitate (*dashed oval*). These cysts have the potential to mimic the erosions of inflammatory arthritis, such as rheumatoid arthritis (RA).

imaging where low to intermediate echo time (TE) imaging (T1, proton density, gradient echo) is routine. Magic angle effect is seen when highly collagenous structures, such as tendons, are oriented at 55° to the magnetic field on these low TE sequences.[40] Due to its course in the wrist,

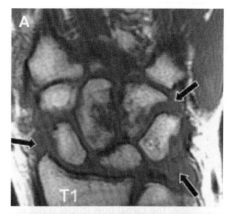

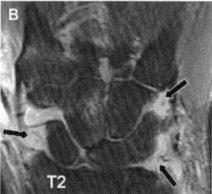

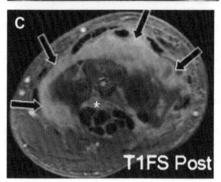

Fig. 12. (*A–C*) A patient with RA. (*A* and *B*) Coronal T1 and T2 sequences, respectively, showing the appearance of extensive pericarpal synovitis (*black block arrows*). Note the edema in the carpal bones on the T2 sequence. (*C*) Axial T1 fat-suppressed image post contrast, demonstrating enhancement of the synovitis, which displaces the extensor tendons (*arrows*) and surrounds the flexor tendons in the carpal tunnel (*asterisk*).

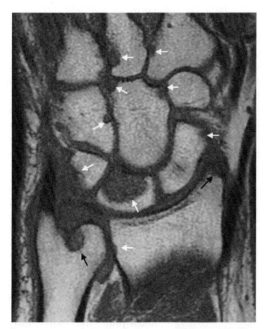

Fig. 11. Coronal T1 image in a patient with known RA. Note numerous erosions (*white arrows*), including those in characteristic locations for RA about the radial styloid and ulnar styloid (*black arrows*).

the extensor pollicis longus (EPL) tendon commonly demonstrates this abnormality.[41] Of the extensor tendons, the extensor carpi ulnaris (ECU) tendon is most commonly tendinotic (**Fig. 17**). Because of the prevalence of ECU tendinopathy, the tendon should be scrutinized, but a nonpathologic increased signal has also been

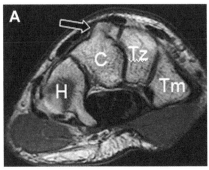
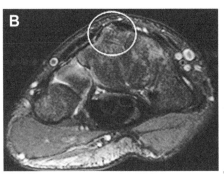
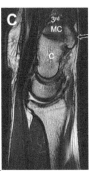

Fig. 13. (*A–C*) A patient with asymptomatic capitate carpal boss. (*A*) Axial T1-weighted image depicting the carpal boss (*black arrow*). Note hamate (H), capitate (C), trapezoid (Tz), and trapezium (Tm). (*B*) Corresponding axial T2 image. The carpal boss (*circle*) is not edematous, and the overlying tendons and soft tissues are not inflamed. (*C*) Sagittal T1 image in the same patient demonstrating the prominent dorsal carpal boss (*black arrow*) at articulation of capitate (C) and third metacarpal base (3rd MC).

noted in the ECU. This increase is thought to be caused by the magic angle effect, based on the spiraling of fibers from the interdigitation of its 2 heads.[41,42]

The ECU is furthermore susceptible to misdiagnosis due to positioning, as pseudosubluxation of the ECU out of its groove has been demonstrated when imaging in supination.[43] Wrist position can be determined by the position of the ECU groove (see **Fig. 17**). When the wrist is imaged in supination the ECU groove is concave dorsal, appearing like a bowl of soup. In the pronated wrist the ECU groove is concave ventral. The neutral wrist is concave medial.[44] Unfortunately, true ECU subluxation is exacerbated with supination as well. Thus, secondary findings are helpful to make the diagnosis of both ECU tendinopathy and instability,[39] as it is unlikely that symptomatic tendon pathology will be present in their absence. Findings present in symptomatic tendons include more intense and diffuse signal alteration as well as morphologic changes in the tendon, for example, thickening or thinning. Intrasubstance signal alteration eventually will approach a fluid

bright signal (interstitial tearing) with progressive injury. Like elsewhere, minimal fluid seen about the wrist tendons may not be symptomatic. This finding has been noted in particular about the extensor carpi radialis brevis (ECRB) and extensor carpi radialis longus (ECRL) tendons. Excess fluid about the tendons when confined by the surrounding tendons sheath is consistent with tenosynovitis (**Fig. 18**).[41]

WRIST LIGAMENTS: TRIANGULAR FIBROCARTILAGE COMPLEX

The triangular fibrocartilage complex (TFCC) is made up of several structures with intricate and blending anatomy. The most significant portion of the TFCC is known as the TFC. This structure stretches from the distal radius abutting the sigmoid notch, across the distal radial ulnar joint (DRUJ), and attaches onto the ulnar styloid.[45] Histologically the TFC is made up of the radioulnar ligament, which is a hammock-like structure that cradles the central fibrocartilaginous disc, leaving only the distal aspect (roof or carpal side) of the

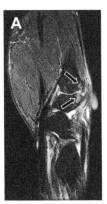
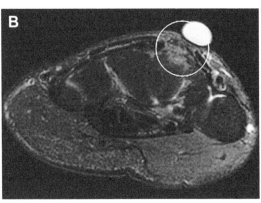

Fig. 14. (*A* and *B*) A patient with a small but symptomatic carpal boss off the trapezium at the CMC joint. (*A*) Sagittal T2-weighted image demonstrating bony edema (*black arrows*) in this patient with carpal boss. (*B*) Corresponding axial T2 image demonstrating soft tissue and marrow edema (*circle*) underlying the soft tissue marker at site of patient's pain. There was no history of trauma.

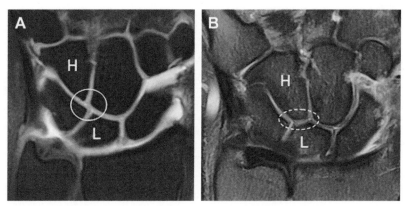

Fig. 15. (A and B) Normal anatomic variation in the lunate (L). (A) Type I lunate (*circle*), which does not have a facet that articulates with the hamate (H). (B) Type II lunate (*dashed oval*), which has a facet that articulates with the hamate (H). There is no MR evidence for chondromalacia, as would be seen with hamatolunate arthrosis.

disc uncovered.[46] The dorsal and volar bands of the radioulnar ligament are commonly described as being 2 separate ligaments, known as the dorsal and volar radioulnar ligaments. The TFC is supported on its volar side by the ulnolunate and ulnotriquetral ligaments, and dorsally by the sheath of the ECU, and blends distally with the traversing ulnar collateral ligament (capsular thickening) to attach to the hamate, triquetrum, and base of the fifth metacarpal.[45]

Palmer[18] originally developed a classification scheme for TFC tears, dividing them by mechanism into traumatic and degenerative tears. MR arthrography may be employed to diagnose and classify such tears, and should include the location, size (length), and thickness (partial or full) of the tear. With regard to location, a tear is either central (radial sided) or peripheral (ulnar sided). The distinction between peripheral and central tear is important, because the former have

a good vascular supply and are thus often repaired, whereas the latter are avascular and are treated with debridement.[47]

On MR imaging the TFC is hypointense, with the exception of its radial and ulnar attachments (**Fig. 19**). A central TFC tear is diagnosed similar to a tear of the meniscus in the knee. Intrasubstance signal alteration that extends to either to the proximal or distal surface is consistent with tear, whereas intrasubstance signal that does not surface is consistent with degeneration. A partial thickness tear contacts only one surface (**Fig. 20**). Contrast communication between the radiocarpal and DRUJ is diagnostic of full-thickness tear. Fluid in the DRUJ is suggestive of full-thickness TFC tear, but may not be diagnostic of tear. It can be likened to fluid in the subacromial subdeltoid bursa, being suggestive of rotator cuff tear while not being indicative of tear. In some instances, reactive fluid may accumulate in both

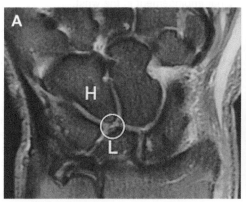
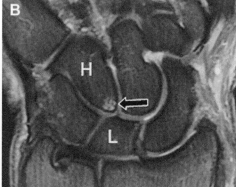

Fig. 16. (A and B) Successive coronal T2 images demonstrating hamatolunate arthrosis in the presence of a type II lunate. (A) Cartilage irregularity at the articulation of the hamate and lunate (*circle*). In B, a black arrow demonstrates edema in the proximal pole of the hamate (H), where it articulates with the lunate (L).

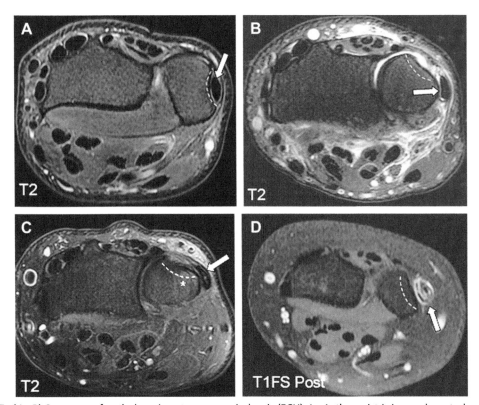

Fig. 17. (*A−D*) Spectrum of pathology in extensor carpi ulnaris (ECU). In *A*, the wrist is imaged neutral position, based on concave medial ECU groove (*curved line*). The ECU (*white arrow*) is normal in signal and is normally situated in the groove. In *B*, the patient was imaged in mild supination, as denoted by the ECU groove being mildly concave dorsally (*curved line*). The ECU (*white arrow*) is subluxed out of its groove with surrounding edema after severe wrist injury. The ECU tendon itself is normal in signal. In *C*, the wrist is imaged in supination and the ECU is subluxed out of its groove (*curved line*). The ECU is mildly tendinotic, demonstrating mild intrasubstance signal alteration (*white arrow*) with reactive edema in the adjacent ulna (*asterisk*). In *D*, the wrist is mildly supinated and the ECU groove (*curved line*) is dysplastic (flat). The ECU is normally positioned in its groove. However, the ECU (*white arrow*) is thickened with intrasubstance and surrounding enhancement, consistent with tendinopathy and tenosynovitis, respectively.

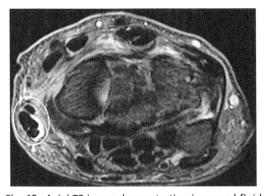

Fig. 18. Axial T2 image demonstrating increased fluid around the first compartment extensor tendons (*circle*), consistent with mild De Quervain tenosynovitis.

locations in the absence of tear, for example, with ulnar impingement in the wrist.

In the presence of even large full-thickness tears, the dorsal and volar radioulnar ligaments often remain intact (**Figs. 21** and **22**). Their presence should not be misdiagnosed as, nor indicate, an intact TFC. Central tears, even large tears, have been shown to increase with age on cadaveric studies, and thus many of them are thought to be degenerative and asymptomatic.[48,49] Hence Gilula and Palmer[50] suggest the term "defect" rather than "tear" may be more appropriate to convey the finding. In contradistinction, traumatic central, full-thickness tears are commonly subtle or "slit-like" and thus may easily be missed (**Fig. 23**).[18] However, a central tear should not be mistakenly diagnosed where the TFC attaches onto the hyaline cartilage of the distal radius,

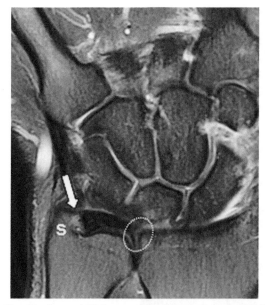

Fig. 19. Coronal T2 image demonstrating the normal appearance of the triangular fibrocartilage (TFC) with the single band variant at the ulnar attachment. Note the smooth, high signal intensity of the hyaline cartilage at the radial attachment (*circle*) and the heterogeneous high signal from fibrous tissue at the ulnar styloid attachment (*white arrow*). S, ulnar styloid.

which is normally hyperintense and may mimic a tear (see **Figs. 19** and **23**).[51]

The ulnar attachment is variable in appearance, and may be a single broad-based attachment (see **Fig. 19**) or 2 distinct laminae attaching to the base and tip of the ulnar styloid (**Fig. 24**).[52] A full-thickness peripheral tear is verified by demonstrating communication of contrast or fluid through the defect (**Fig. 25**). However, not all tears

are full thickness, and the ulnar attachment of the TFC is also fraught with more potential pitfalls than is the radial attachment. Zanetti and colleagues[53] have shown that symptomatic noncommunicating (partial thickness) defects are common at the ulnar attachment. Single-compartment arthrography (radiocarpal injection) is suboptimal in evaluating these partial thickness defects because, as expected, they do not demonstrate direct communication between the radiocarpal compartment and DRUJ. Accurate diagnosis is further challenging because the ulnar attachment is normally increased in signal. False-positive peripheral tears have been reported secondary to increased signal at the striated peripheral attachment,[54] signal alteration from fibrous connective tissue between the 2 laminae,[51] and with volume averaging from surrounding fluid signal (focal synovitis).[55] Given these challenges, dual-compartment MR arthrography is recommended, with injection into both the radiocarpal and DRUJ to reduce missed noncommunicating tears and to diminish the likelihood of false-positive tears.

WRIST LIGAMENTS: SL AND LT

The extrinsic ligaments link the radius and ulna to carpal bones and the intrinsic wrist ligaments link carpal bones to one another.[56] The distal intrinsic ligaments are rarely studied and do not seal off the midcarpal joint from the carpal metacarpal (CMC) joint.[57] This appearance is often demonstrated with the midcarpal injection in arthrography, as contrast extravasates at the CMC with joint filling. The commonly studied SL and LT ligaments seal off the radiocarpal joint from the midcarpal joint proximally.[58] These ligaments are U-shaped, with ligamentous dorsal and volar bands and a central membranous (proximal)

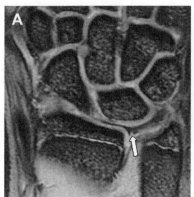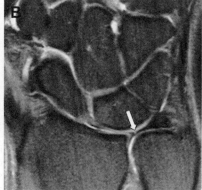

Fig. 20. (*A* and *B*) Partial-thickness tears abutting the radial attachment of the TFC. (*A*) Coronal T2* sequence showing a partial thickness central tear of the TFC involving the proximal surface (*white arrow*). (*B*) Coronal T1 arthrographic sequence showing partial thickness distal tear of TFC (*white arrow*).

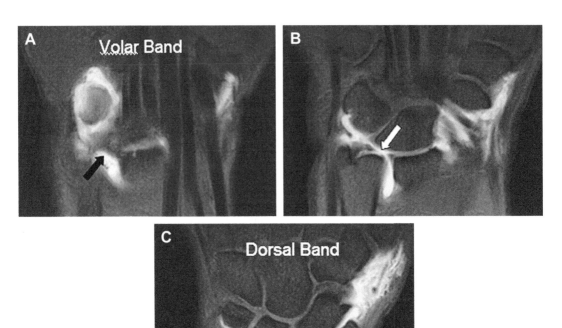

Fig. 21. (A–C) Nonsequential coronal T1 arthrographic images from volar to dorsal demonstrating a central full-thickness TFC tear. (A) Intact volar band of the radioulnar ligament (*black arrow*). (B) Contrast extending through a full-thickness TFC tear (*large white arrow*). (C) Intact dorsal band of the radioulnar ligament (*black arrow*).

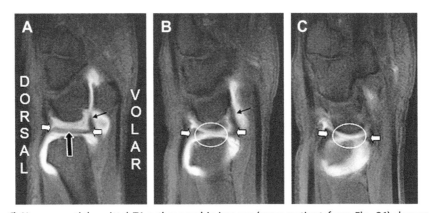

Fig. 22. (A–C) Nonsequential sagittal T1 arthrographic images (same patient from **Fig. 21**) demonstrating the central full-thickness TFC tear. A is toward the ulnar side of the TFC and demonstrates the intact central fibrocartilaginous disc (*black block arrow*) as well as intact dorsal and volar bands of the radioulnar ligament (*white arrows*). B is 2 cuts radially, demonstrating the intact dorsal and ulnar bands (*white arrows*) with marked thinning of the central fibrocartilaginous disk (*circle*). C is 2 cuts radially, abutting the radial attachment of the TFC. The dorsal and ulnar bands (*white arrows*) are intact, but there is contrast traversing the full-thickness central tear of the fibrocartilaginous disk (*circle*). Note intact ulnolunate ligament (*black line arrow*) in A and B.

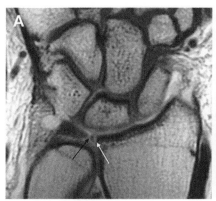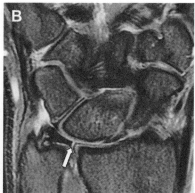

Fig. 23. (*A* and *B*) Traumatic central full-thickness tears. (*A*) Coronal nonfat-suppressed T1 arthrographic image in a 12-year-old girl with an acute injury demonstrating a thin full-thickness tear (*black arrow*), which is immediately adjacent to the radial attachment of the TFC. Note adjacent normal hyaline cartilage at the radial attachment of the TFC (*white arrow*). (*B*) Nonarthrographic coronal T2 sequence in an 18-year-old man with an acute injury demonstrating a central full-thickness tear (*white arrow*).

band.[58–60] Wrist stability is determined by the complex interplay between intrinsic and extrinsic wrist ligaments.[61] The dorsal aspect of the SL ligament and the volar band of the LT ligament should be scrutinized, because they are thought to be the most important component of each ligament in maintaining wrist stability.[51,62,63] Like TFC tears, SL and LT tears increase with age and may be asymptomatic, particularly when involving the membranous portion of each ligament.[49,63]

Depiction of ligamentous injury on MR imaging, even with arthrography, presents a unique challenge given the morphology and small size of these ligaments.[64] Using the axial and coronal planes together best depicts the components of the SL and LT ligaments. The hypointense dorsal, volar, and membranous bands of both ligaments may all be seen in the coronal plane (**Fig. 26**). The axial plane does not well evaluate the membranous band of the SL or LT ligament. However, it does often nicely depict the dorsal and volar bands of the SL ligament (**Fig. 27**) because they are commonly in the conventional axial imaging plane. The axial plane may not evaluate the dorsal and volar bands of the LT ligament as well as the SL ligament, because the traditional axial plane commonly runs obliquely through this more diminutive ligament (see **Fig. 26**B). Obtaining the MR examination in ulnar or radial deviation as well as tailoring the axial images to the plane of the suspected ligament injury has been shown to be helpful in depicting these ligaments.[65] A tear of any or all of the 3 components is diagnosed by visualizing partial or complete ligamentous discontinuity with bridging fluid or contrast signal (**Figs. 28–30**).[47] When possible, it is helpful for presurgical planning to describe which band is torn, as well as which side of the ligament is torn. For example, knowing that the dorsal band of the scapholunate ligament is torn from its attachment off the scaphoid (rather than a midsubstance tear

Fig. 24. Coronal protein density (PD) sequence demonstrating dual-band variant of the ulnar attachment of the TFC. Note the attachment to the base of the ulnar styloid (*black arrow*) and to the tip of the ulnar styloid (*white arrow*). The normal intervening fibrofatty tissue is intermediate in signal intensity.

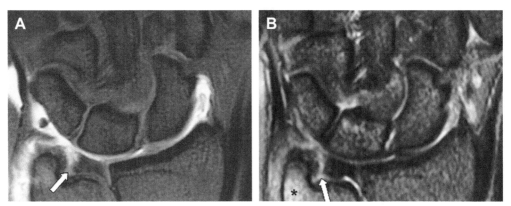

Fig. 25. (*A* and *B*) Coronal images showing a peripheral full-thickness TFC tear. (*A*) T1 arthrographic image showing contrast extending through the full-thickness peripheral tear (*white arrow*). (*B*) T2-weighted gradient echo image in the same patient demonstrating fluid traversing the peripheral full-thickness tear (*white arrow*) with edema in the ulnar styloid (*asterisk*).

or tear of the lunate attachment) is helpful in planning which arthroscopic portal is optimal for reconstruction. Intrasubstance signal alteration can be seen within both ligaments and should not be misinterpreted as a tear, nor should intermediate intensity signal alteration at the membranous attachments, which insert onto hyaline cartilage.[47,66,67] On axial imaging the traversing extrinsic ligaments should not be mistaken for intact dorsal and volar bands (see **Fig. 29**).

WRIST NERVES

MR imaging is used to assess for peripheral nerve entrapment throughout the body. In the wrist, MR imaging may be prescribed to evaluate for median or ulnar nerve compression. The diagnosis of nerve entrapment is commonly made using a combination of clinical and electrodiagnostic findings, and are treated with therapies aimed at

decreasing pressure caused by mass compression or inflammation.[68] MR is typically employed when extrinsic compression from mass is suspected, and in patients with persistent symptoms despite empiric treatment.[69] Both the median and ulnar nerves are normally isointense to slightly hyperintense to muscle on T2 fat-suppressed sequences. A combination of axial and fluid-sensitive sequences (for example, nonfat-suppressed T1 and T2 fat-suppressed or short-tau inversion recovery) together nicely portray the normal anatomy, as well as demonstrate associated inflammation, mass, or other pathologic changes. Knowledge of the normal anatomy in Guyon's canal and the carpal tunnel is imperative so as not to misdiagnose normal variants as pathology.

The most common wrist neuropathy is carpal tunnel syndrome (CTS), which is compressive neuropathy of the median nerve. The contents of

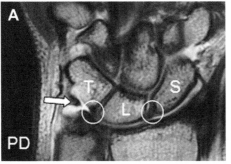
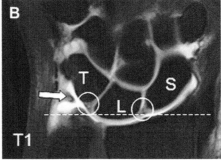

Fig. 26. (*A* and *B*) Normal appearance of the scapholunate (SL) and lunotriquetral (LT) ligaments on PD and T1-weighted images, respectively. On both images the SL ligament is circled between the scaphoid (S) and lunate (L). The LT ligament is circled between the lunate (L) and triquetrum (T). Note the normal meniscal homologue (*white arrows*). Dashed line in *B* shows the conventional axial plane of imaging, which closely follows the axis of the SL ligament, but not the LT ligament.

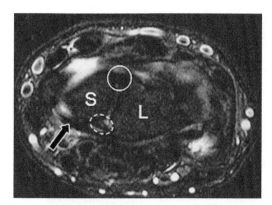

Fig. 27. T2-weighted gradient echo nonarthrographic axial image demonstrating the normal dorsal band (*solid circle*) and volar band (*dashed oval*) of the SL ligament. The overlying radiolunotriquetral ligament (*black arrow*) is intimate with the volar band and should not be mistaken as the volar band of the SL ligament. L, lunate; S, scaphoid.

the carpal tunnel include the median nerve and 9 flexor tendons.[70] The carpal bones form the floor of the carpal tunnel. The volar aspect of the proximal carpal tunnel is bound by the flexor retinaculum and transverse carpal ligament, which stretch across the pisiform and scaphoid. Distally, this fibrous band extends between the hook of the hamate and tubercle of the trapezium.[70,71] MR findings that may be present in the setting of CTS include size and signal changes in the median nerve, bowing of the retinaculum, or pathologic processes that produce a mass effect in the carpal tunnel (**Fig. 31**).[72,73] Typical changes observed in the median nerve include edema, thickening proximal to the carpal tunnel, and flattening within the carpal tunnel.[69] The diagnostic utility of these

findings is controversial because they are not sensitive for CTS, particularly when present alone. Nor are they specific, as size and signal changes of the median nerve can be seen in the absence of CTS.[74] Thus, the aforementioned MR findings should be correlated with clinical symptoms so as not to overcall CTS. Care must also be taken not to misdiagnose known anomalies such as bifid median nerve with or without a persistent median artery, neuroma, and lipohamartoma as CTS (**Figs. 32 and 33**).[75]

The causes of ulnar neuropathy are many. Microrepetitive trauma is often the culprit, particularly in those with recreational or occupational vibration exposure. Examples of those at risk include cyclists (handlebar palsy) and construction workers.[76] The ulnar nerve and vessels are encased by fat and pass though the wrist via Guyon's canal, a fibro-osseous tunnel beginning at the base of the pisiform extending through the hamate, with 3 anatomic zones based on standard branching of the ulnar nerve.[77,78] The shape of Guyon's canal is variable, but is generally triangular proximally at its inlet at the level of the pisiform (Zone I). The mid tunnel (Zone II) becomes more oval shaped, and is the typical location of bifurcation of the ulnar nerve into its sensory and motor branches. The distal canal is located at the level of the hamate, where it flattens out into a biconvex or discoid shape. It is here in Zone III that Guyon's canal becomes separated by the fibrous arch or muscle belly of the flexor digiti minimi brevis muscle into dorsal and palmar channels, which contain the motor and sensory branches of the ulnar nerve, respectively.[77]

The MR findings associated with ulnar nerve compression in Guyon's canal are less extensively

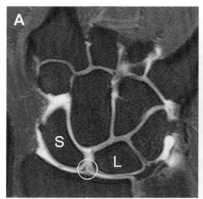
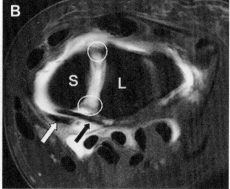

Fig. 28. (*A and B*) Partial tear of the SL ligament. (*A*) Coronal T1 arthrographic image demonstrating contrast extending across a full-thickness tear of the membranous portion of the SL ligament (*circle*). (*B*) Axial T1 arthrographic image in the same patient showing the intact dorsal band (*circle*) and volar band (*oval*) of the SL ligament. Note the overlying or radiolunotriquetral (*black arrow*) and radioscapholunate (*white arrow*) ligaments, which are separated from the volar band of SL with joint distension. L, lunate; S, scaphoid.

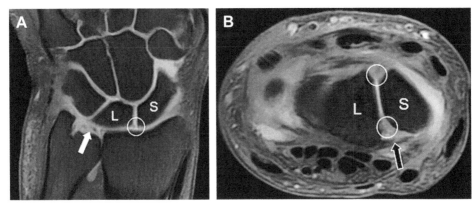

Fig. 29. (*A* and *B*) Complete SL ligament tear. (*A*) Coronal T1 arthrographic image depicting the torn membranous band of the SL ligament (*circle*). Note the severely macerated TFC (*white arrow*). (*B*) Axial T1 arthrographic image demonstrating the disrupted dorsal and volar bands of SL. Note overlying and intact radiolunotriquetral ligament (*black arrow*), which should not be mistaken for the intact volar band of the SL ligament. L, lunate; S, scaphoid.

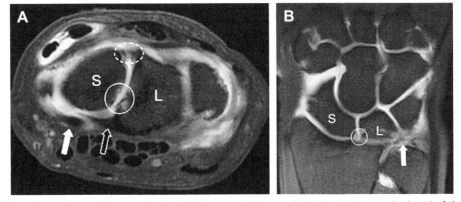

Fig. 30. (*A* and *B*) SL ligament tear. (*A*) Axial T1 arthrographic image depicting the torn volar band of the SL ligament (*circle*). The dorsal band of the SL is intact (*dashed oval*). Note overlying radiolunotriquetral (*black arrow*) and radioscapholunate (*white arrow*) ligaments. (*B*) Coronal T1 arthrographic image in the same patient image demonstrating corresponding SL tear (*white circle*). Note macerated TFC (*white arrow*). L, lunate; S, scaphoid.

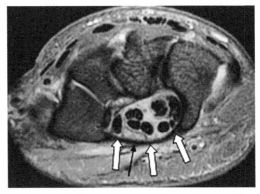

Fig. 31. Axial T2 sequence in a patient with flexor tenosynovitis causing carpal tunnel syndrome. Note the fluid surrounding all the flexor tendons in the carpal tunnel, the bowed flexor retinaculum (*white block arrows*), and the enlarged and edematous median nerve (*black block arrow*).

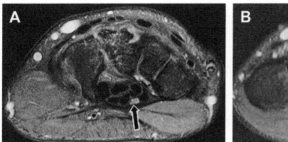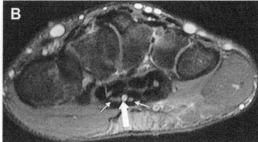

Fig. 32. (A and B) Anatomic variation of the median nerve. (A) Normal median nerve (black arrow), which normally demonstrates mild T2 hyperintensity with fasciculations (black arrow). In B, one can appreciate the 2 bundles of a bifid median nerve (white line arrows) with a centrally situated persistent median artery (white block arrow).

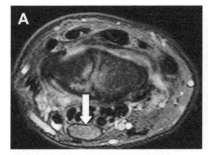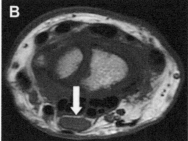

Fig. 33. (A and B) T2- and T1-weighted images, respectively, demonstrating a neuroma of the median nerve (white arrows), located just proximal to carpal tunnel. A lipohamartoma would appear similar but would demonstrate internal fat signal on the nonfat-suppressed T1 image. Marked enlargement of the median nerve with carpal tunnel syndrome could appear similar to a neuroma.

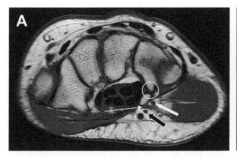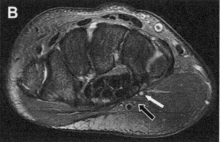

Fig. 34. (A and B) A patient with ulnar neuropathy. (A) Axial T1 image demonstrating an ununited hook of the hamate fracture (circle). The normal bifurcation of Guyon's canal displays the dorsal (motor) branch of the ulnar nerve (white block arrow) and volar (sensory) branch of the ulnar nerve (black block arrow). The dorsal and ulnar nerves are separated by the flexor digiti minimi brevis muscle (white line arrow). (B) Corresponding T2-weighted image demonstrating mild hyperintensity within the motor branch of the ulnar nerve (white block arrow) with minimal surrounding edema. Compare with the normal signal intensity of the sensory branch of the ulnar nerve (black arrow). The patient's symptoms improved after resection of the hook of the hamate.

studied than CTS, perhaps because of a combination of its small size relative to the median nerve and the lack of success in finding diagnostic criteria on MR for CTS. As with median nerve neuropathy, MR imaging is best employed to look for mass compression of the ulnar nerve, which can be secondary to vascular anomalies (varices or aneurysm), soft tissue neoplasm, ganglion cysts, fibrous bands, hamate anomalies, and anomalous muscle.[76,79–82] With regard to ulnar neuropathy, nonunion or malunion of a hook of the hamate fracture may be the cause of the patient's symptoms (**Fig. 34**). Chronic fractures that are not highlighted by edema, as well as small cortical bone fragments, may be subtle and therefore may be initially overlooked on MR imaging (see **Figs. 4** and **34**). Correlation with radiographs and MR imaging protocols that obtain some nonfat-suppressed sequences are helpful in making these diagnoses.

WRIST IMAGING: RADIOLOGIC REPORT

In the past, MR imaging of the wrist was only useful in diagnosing pathology such as occult carpal fractures. Recently improved technology has taken MR imaging of the wrist mainstream. When presented with the aforementioned information, the radiologist should have concluded that general protocols employed for accurate diagnosis of pathology in large joints may not be suitable for some wrist imaging. Accurate depiction of the diminutive anatomic structures of the wrist may require close surveillance as they are acquired, at least initially. When generating the radiologic report, the consulting radiologist must be aware of the limitations of wrist imaging, general MR imaging pitfalls applicable to the wrist, asymptomatic anatomic variation that may be misdiagnosed as pathology, and anatomic variation that predisposes the patient to specific pathologic processes. This information makes or confirms the diagnosis and thus helps determine the appropriate treatment. In those instances where surgery is needed, the information is critical for orthopedic colleagues in determining the need for, type of, and timing of surgery.

REFERENCES

1. Greenspan A. Orthopedic imaging: a practical approach. Philadelphia: Lippincott Williams & Wilkins; 2004.
2. Yang Z, Mann FA, Gilula LA, et al. Scaphopisocapitate alignment: criterion to establish a neutral lateral view of the wrist. Radiology 1997;205(3):865–9.
3. Jedlinski A, Kauer JM, Jonsson K. X-ray evaluation of the true neutral position of the wrist: the groove for extensor carpi ulnaris as a landmark. J Hand Surg Am 1995;20(3):511–2.
4. Levis CM, Yang Z, Gilula LA. Validation of the extensor carpi ulnaris groove as a predictor for the recognition of standard posteroanterior radiographs of the wrist. J Hand Surg Am 2002;27(2):252–7.
5. Zlatkin MB, Chao PC, Osterman AL, et al. Chronic wrist pain: evaluation with high-resolution MR imaging. Radiology 1989;173(3):723–9.
6. Gilula LA, Weeks PM. Post-traumatic ligamentous instabilities of the wrist. Radiology 1978;129(3): 641–51.
7. Zanetti M, Hodler J, Gilula LA. Assessment of dorsal or ventral intercalated segmental instability configurations of the wrist: reliability of sagittal MR images. Radiology 1998;206(2):339–45.
8. Cerezal L, Abascal F, Garcia-Valtuille R, et al. Wrist MR arthrography: how, why, when. Radiol Clin North Am 2005;43(4):709–31, viii.
9. Hodge JC, Gilula LA. Imaging of the wrist and hand. J South Orthop Assoc 1996;5(4):292–304.
10. Epner RA, Bowers WH, Guilford WB. Ulnar variance—the effect of wrist positioning and roentgen filming technique. J Hand Surg Am 1982;7(3):298–305.
11. Friedman SL, Palmer AK, Short WH, et al. The change in ulnar variance with grip. J Hand Surg Am 1993;18(4):713–6.
12. Palmer AK, Glisson RR, Werner FW. Ulnar variance determination. J Hand Surg Am 1982;7(4):376–9.
13. Friedman SL, Palmer AK. The ulnar impaction syndrome. Hand Clin 1991;7(2):295–310.
14. Tomaino MM. Ulnar impaction syndrome in the ulnar negative and neutral wrist. Diagnosis and pathoanatomy. J Hand Surg Br 1998;23(6):754–7.
15. Escobedo EM, Bergman AG, Hunter JC. MR imaging of ulnar impaction. Skeletal Radiol 1995; 24(2):85–90.
16. Imaeda T, Nakamura R, Shionoya K, et al. Ulnar impaction syndrome: MR imaging findings. Radiology 1996;201(2):495–500.
17. Cerezal L, del Piñal F, Abascal F, et al. Imaging findings in ulnar-sided wrist impaction syndromes. Radiographics 2002;22(1):105–21.
18. Palmer AK. Triangular fibrocartilage complex lesions: a classification. J Hand Surg Am 1989;14(4): 594–606.
19. Tomaino MM, Elfar J. Ulnar impaction syndrome. Hand Clin 2005;21(4):567–75.
20. Bell MJ, Hill RJ, McMurtry RY. Ulnar impingement syndrome. J Bone Joint Surg Br 1985;67(1): 126–9.
21. McQueen F, Ostergaard M, Peterfy C, et al. Pitfalls in scoring MR images of rheumatoid arthritis wrist and metacarpophalangeal joints. Ann Rheum Dis 2005; 64(Suppl 1):i48–55.

22. Ejbjerg B, Narvestad E, Rostrup E, et al. Magnetic resonance imaging of wrist and finger joints in healthy subjects occasionally shows changes resembling erosions and synovitis as seen in rheumatoid arthritis. Arthritis Rheum 2004;50(4): 1097–106.

23. Narvaez JA, Narvaez J, De Lama E, et al. MR imaging of early rheumatoid arthritis. Radiographics 2010;30(1):143–63 [discussion: 163–5].

24. Artz TD, Posch JL. The carpometacarpal boss. J Bone Joint Surg Am 1973;55(4):747–52.

25. Fusi S, Watson HK, Cuono CB. The carpal boss: a 20-year review of operative management. J Hand Surg Br 1995;20(3):405–8.

26. Conway WF, Destouet JM, Gilula LA, et al. The carpal boss: an overview of radiographic evaluation. Radiology 1985;156(1):29–31.

27. Cuone CB, Watson HK. The carpal boss: surgical treatment and etiological considerations. Plast Reconstr Surg 1979;63(1):88–93.

28. Park MJ, Namdari S, Weiss A. The carpal boss: review of diagnosis and treatment. J Hand Surg 2008;33(3):446–9.

29. Vermeulen GM, de With MC, Bleys RL, et al. Carpal boss: effect of wedge excision depth on third carpometacarpal joint stability. J Hand Surg Am 2009;34(1):7–13.

30. Viegas SF, Wagner K, Patterson R, et al. Medial (hamate) facet of the lunate. J Hand Surg 1990; 15(4):564–71.

31. Viegas SF, Patterson RM, Hokanson JA, et al. Wrist anatomy: incidence, distribution, and correlation of anatomic variations, tears, and arthrosis. J Hand Surg 1993;18(3):463–75.

32. Pfirrmann CW, Theumann NH, Chung CB, et al. The hamatolunate facet: characterization and association with cartilage lesions—magnetic resonance arthrography and anatomic correlation in cadaveric wrists. Skeletal Radiol 2002;31(8):451–6.

33. Nakamura K, Patterson RM, Moritomo H, et al. Type I versus type II lunates: ligament anatomy and presence of arthrosis. J Hand Surg 2001;26(3):428–36.

34. Malik A, Schweitzer M, Culp R, et al. MR imaging of the type II lunate bone: frequency, extent, and associated findings. Am J Roentgenol 1999;173(2): 335–8.

35. Zanetti M, Saupe N, Nagy L. Role of MR imaging in chronic wrist pain. Eur Radiol 2007;17(4):927–38.

36. Rubenstein J, Li J, Majumdar S, et al. Image resolution and signal-to-noise ratio requirements for MR imaging of degenerative cartilage. Am J Roentgenol 1997;169(4):1089–96.

37. Thurston AJ, Stanley JK. Hamato-lunate impingement: an uncommon cause of ulnar-sided wrist pain. Arthroscopy 2000;16(5):540–4.

38. Harley BJ, Werner FW, Boles SD, et al. Arthroscopic resection of arthrosis of the proximal hamate:

a clinical and biomechanical study. J Hand Surg Am 2004;29(4):661–7.

39. Bencardino JT. MR imaging of tendon lesions of the hand and wrist. Magn Reson Imaging Clin N Am 2004;12(2):333–47, vii.

40. Fullerton GD, Cameron IL, Ord VA. Orientation of tendons in the magnetic field and its effect on T2 relaxation times. Radiology 1985;155(2):433–5.

41. Timins ME, O'Connell SE, Erickson SJ, et al. MR imaging of the wrist: normal findings that may simulate disease. Radiographics 1996;16(5): 987–95.

42. Tountas CP, Bergman RA. Anatomic variations of the upper extremity. New York: Churchill Livingston; 1993.

43. Pfirrmann CW, Theumann NH, Chung CB, et al. What happens to the triangular fibrocartilage complex during pronation and supination of the forearm? Analysis of its morphology and diagnostic assessment with MR arthrography. Skeletal Radiol 2001;30(12):677–85.

44. Stoller DW, Li AE, Lichtman DM, et al. The wrist and hand. In: Stoller DW, editor. Magnetic resonance imaging in orthopaedics and sports medicine. Baltimore (MD): Lippincott, Williams, and Wilkins; 2007. p. 1674.

45. Palmer AK, Werner FW. The triangular fibrocartilage complex of the wrist—anatomy and function. J Hand Surg Am 1981;6(2):153–62.

46. Nakamura T, Yabe Y. Histological anatomy of the triangular fibrocartilage complex of the human wrist. Ann Anat 2000;182(6):567–72.

47. Zlatkin MB, Rosner J. MR imaging of ligaments and triangular fibrocartilage complex of the wrist. Magn Reson Imaging Clin N Am 2004;12(2):301–31, vi–vii.

48. Mikic ZD. Age changes in the triangular fibrocartilage of the wrist joint. J Anat 1978;126(Pt 2):367–84.

49. Lee DH, Dickson KF, Bradley EL. The incidence of wrist interosseous ligament and triangular fibrocartilage articular disc disruptions: a cadaveric study. J Hand Surg Am 2004;29(4):676–84.

50. Gilula LA, Palmer AK. Is it possible to diagnose a tear at arthrography or MR imaging? Radiology 1993;187(2):582.

51. Timins ME, Jahnke JP, Krah SF, et al. MR imaging of the major carpal stabilizing ligaments: normal anatomy and clinical examples. Radiographics 1995;15(3):575–87.

52. Totterman SM, Miller RJ. Triangular fibrocartilage complex: normal appearance on coronal three-dimensional gradient-recalled-echo MR images. Radiology 1995;195(2):521–7.

53. Zanetti M, Linkous MD, Gilula LA, et al. Characteristics of triangular fibrocartilage defects in symptomatic and contralateral asymptomatic wrists. Radiology 2000;216(3):840–5.

54. Oneson SR, Timins ME, Scales LM, et al. MR imaging diagnosis of triangular fibrocartilage pathology with arthroscopic correlation. AJR Am J Roentgenol 1997;168(6):1513–8.

55. Haims AH, Schweitzer ME, Morrison WB, et al. Limitations of MR imaging in the diagnosis of peripheral tears of the triangular fibrocartilage of the wrist. AJR Am J Roentgenol 2002;178(2):419–22.

56. Taleisnik J. Current concepts review. Carpal instability. J Bone Joint Surg Am 1988;70(8):1262–8.

57. Bogumill G. Anatomy of the wrist. In: Lichtman DM, editor. The wrist and its disorders. Philadelphia: W.B. Saunders; 1997. p. 34–48.

58. Berger RA. The gross and histologic anatomy of the scapholunate interosseous ligament. J Hand Surg Am 1996;21(2):170–8.

59. Berger RA. The anatomy of the ligaments of the wrist and distal radioulnar joints. Clin Orthop Relat Res 2001;383:32–40.

60. Pfirrmann CW, Zanetti M. Variants, pitfalls and asymptomatic findings in wrist and hand imaging. Eur J Radiol 2005;56(3):286–95.

61. Theumann NH, Etechami G, Duvoisin B, et al. Association between extrinsic and intrinsic carpal ligament injuries at MR arthrography and carpal instability at radiography: initial observations. Radiology 2006;238(3):950–7.

62. Mitsuyasu H, Patterson RM, Shah MA, et al. The role of the dorsal intercarpal ligament in dynamic and static scapholunate instability. J Hand Surg Am 2004;29(2):279–88.

63. Linkous MD, Pierce SD, Gilula LA. Scapholunate ligamentous communicating defects in symptomatic and asymptomatic wrists: characteristics. Radiology 2000;216(3):846–50.

64. Manton GL, Schweitzer ME, Weishaupt D, et al. Partial interosseous ligament tears of the wrist: difficulty in utilizing either primary or secondary MRI signs. J Comput Assist Tomogr 2001;25(5):671–6.

65. Gheno R, Buck FM, Nico MA, et al. Differences between radial and ulnar deviation of the wrist in the study of the intrinsic intercarpal ligaments: magnetic resonance imaging and gross anatomic inspection in cadavers. Skeletal Radiol 2010;39(8):799–805.

66. Smith DK. Scapholunate interosseous ligament of the wrist: MR appearances in asymptomatic volunteers and arthrographically normal wrists. Radiology 1994;192(1):217–21.

67. Smith DK, Snearly WN. Lunotriquetral interosseous ligament of the wrist: MR appearances in asymptomatic volunteers and arthrographically normal wrists. Radiology 1994;191(1):199–202.

68. Katz JN, Simmons BP. Clinical practice. Carpal tunnel syndrome. N Engl J Med 2002;346(23):1807–12.

69. Bordalo-Rodrigues M, Amin P, Rosenberg ZS. MR imaging of common entrapment neuropathies at the wrist. Magn Reson Imaging Clin N Am 2004;12(2):265–79, vi.

70. Mesgarzadeh M, Schneck CD, Bonakdarpour A. Carpal tunnel: MR imaging. Part I. Normal anatomy. Radiology 1989;171(3):743–8.

71. Martinoli C, Bianchi S, Gandolfo N, et al. US of nerve entrapments in osteofibrous tunnels of the upper and lower limbs. Radiographics 2000;20(Spec No):S199–213 [discussion: S213–7].

72. Mesgarzadeh M, Schneck CD, Bonakdarpour A, et al. Carpal tunnel: MR imaging. Part II. Carpal tunnel syndrome. Radiology 1989;171(3):749–54.

73. Monagle K, Dai G, Chu A, et al. Quantitative MR imaging of carpal tunnel syndrome. AJR Am J Roentgenol 1999;172(6):1581–6.

74. Radack DM, Schweitzer ME, Taras J. Carpal tunnel syndrome: are the MR findings a result of population selection bias? AJR Am J Roentgenol 1997;169(6):1649–53.

75. Lanz U. Anatomical variations of the median nerve in the carpal tunnel. J Hand Surg Am 1977;2(1):44–53.

76. Blum AG, Zabel JP, Kohlmann R, et al. Pathologic conditions of the hypothenar eminence: evaluation with multidetector CT and MR imaging. Radiographics 2006;26(4):1021–44.

77. Zeiss J, Jakab E, Khimji T, et al. The ulnar tunnel at the wrist (Guyon's canal): normal MR anatomy and variants. AJR Am J Roentgenol 1992;158(5):1081–5.

78. Gross MS, Gelberman RH. The anatomy of the distal ulnar tunnel. Clin Orthop Relat Res 1985;196:238–47.

79. Yoshii S, Ikeda K, Murakami H. Ulnar nerve compression secondary to ulnar artery true aneurysm at Guyon's canal. J Neurosurg Sci 1999;43(4):295–7.

80. Greene MH, Hadied AM. Bipartite hamulus with ulnar tunnel syndrome—case report and literature review. J Hand Surg Am 1981;6(6):605–9.

81. Ruocco MJ, Walsh JJ, Jackson JP. MR imaging of ulnar nerve entrapment secondary to an anomalous wrist muscle. Skeletal Radiol 1998;27(4):218–21.

82. Murata K, Shih JT, Tsai TM. Causes of ulnar tunnel syndrome: a retrospective study of 31 subjects. J Hand Surg Am 2003;28(4):647–51.

MR Imaging of the Hip: Normal Anatomic Variants and Imaging Pitfalls

David F. DuBois, MD, Imran M. Omar, MD*

KEYWORDS
- Labral anatomy • MRI • Arthrography • Labral tears

MR imaging of the hip is one of the most common musculoskeletal MR imaging studies performed today to assess for occult fractures, acetabular labral tears, hyaline cartilage loss, and musculotendinous injuries. Several developmental variations are seen in the hip, which can be mistaken for disease or potentially even contribute to the development of a pathologic condition. As in any imaging study, it is important to be cognizant of these variations as well as associated findings that help distinguish between true abnormality and developmental variation when interpreting an MR image of the hip. This article describes the numerous variants of the hip that are frequently seen on arthrographic and nonarthrographic MR imaging examinations.

LABRAL ANATOMY

The acetabular labrum is a fibrocartilaginous horseshoe-shaped structure along the anterior, superior, and posterior margins of the acetabular rim. Unlike the knee menisci, which have a load-bearing and cushioning function, and the glenoid labrum, which helps to deepen the glenoid fossa and improve glenohumeral contiguity, the acetabular labrum primarily seals the margins of the articular hyaline cartilage to prevent premature cartilage loss. However, repetitive impingement and labral tears are a frequent cause of hip pain. Tears occur most commonly in the anterior superior quadrant of the labrum.[1] As a result, evaluation of the labrum to detect abnormalities before the

onset of cartilage loss is among the most common indications for imaging of the hip. Occasionally, patients may have asymptomatic labral tears or developmental variations that mimic labral pathology. These patients may benefit from MR arthrography, which distends joint recesses and increases intra-articular pressure, thereby allowing detection of smaller labral tears. Simultaneous intra-articular local anesthetic injection may also be useful to help distinguish between symptomatic and asymptomatic labral tears or developmental variations.

On imaging, the labrum is usually triangular and slightly thicker posterosuperiorly than anteriorly.[2] The labrum usually has a low signal intensity on all routinely used pulse sequences, particularly on more heavily T2-weighted sequences with longer echo times (TE). Several variations in the morphology and imaging appearance of the acetabular labrum can mimic pathologic conditions and lead to ineffective treatment.

Labral tears or detachments can be seen on nonarthrographic MR studies with linear fluid signal tracking into the labral substance or undermining the labral attachment to the acetabular rim. Many tears have intrasubstance high signal on T2-weighted or proton density sequences, with surface irregularity and irregularity of the adjacent hyaline cartilage. Tears can be diagnosed on MR arthrography by visualizing injected contrast material extending into the labrum or through the labrum/acetabulum junction. In more advanced cases, there may be blunting of the labrum, with

Department of Radiology, Northwestern University Feinberg School of Medicine, 676 North Saint Clair Street, Suite 800, Chicago, IL, 60611, USA
* Corresponding author.
E-mail address: imran.omar@nmff.org

Magn Reson Imaging Clin N Am 18 (2010) 663–674
doi:10.1016/j.mric.2010.09.003
1064-9689/10/$ — see front matter © 2010 Elsevier Inc. All rights reserved.

loss of the normal triangular morphology. Often there is a paralabral cyst with a neck arising either from the labrum itself or from the labro-osseous interface that is commonly seen in association with labral tears.[3]

INTERMEDIATE LABRUM SIGNAL

Increased signal within the labrum can be a normal finding, particularly on shorter TE pulse sequences such as T1-weighted or proton density techniques. Hodler and colleagues[4] compared MR images of the hip with histologic findings in cadavers and found that abnormal signal in the acetabular labrum correlated poorly with histologic signs of degeneration. In a study of 52 hips in 46 asymptomatic volunteers, Cotten and colleagues[5] found areas of intermediate or high labral signal intensity in 58% of hips on T1- and proton density–weighted spin echo images in nonarthrographic studies. Intralabral signal was globular, linear, or curvilinear and was located in the superior (87%), posterior (21%), and anterior (8%) labrum. In their study, the abnormal signal was sometimes seen extending to the capsular and/or articular surfaces of the labrum, thus mimicking labral tears in these asymptomatic patients. Although many of these abnormalities resolved on more heavily T2-weighted sequences, intermediate signal persisted in 12% of labra on both T2-weighted conventional spin echo and fast spin echo images. Thus, one should be cautious when relying exclusively on intrasubstance signal alterations to detect labral tears.

LABRAL SHAPE

The acetabular labrum is normally triangular in cross section, with the lateral part forming the tip and the broader base attached to the bony acetabulum. The labrum is normally thinner anteriorly and thicker superiorly and posteriorly.[2,6] However, there is a variability in labrum shape in asymptomatic subjects. In their study of MR imaging examinations on 200 asymptomatic hips, Lecouvet and colleagues[7] found the classic triangular labral shape in only 66% of cases, with a round shape in 11% and a flat shape in 9%. They also reported that the prevalence of a triangular labrum decreases with age.

HYPOPLASIA OF LABRUM

The Buford complex in the shoulder is a well-described normal variant, where there is hypoplasia of the anterosuperior glenoid labrum with an associated enlarged middle glenohumeral ligament.[8] There is debate as to whether a similar phenomenon occurs in the acetabular labrum. Cotten and colleagues[5] reported that the anterosuperior labrum was absent in 10% of asymptomatic hips. Lecouvet and colleagues[7] described an increased incidence of labral nonvisualization with increasing age in asymptomatic patients. In a study of 40 symptomatic patients and 6 cadaveric hip joint specimens using MRI arthrography followed by cryosectioning, Czerny and colleagues[2] found that the labrum was present in all patients and specimens, with no areas of focal absence. Dinauer and colleagues[9] found no instance of an absent portion of the labrum in 58 patients. The finding of absent labral segments may be because of close proximity of the labrum and capsule, precluding resolution of the 2 separate structures.[6] The authors opine that until more work is done that supports focal absence of the labrum is a normal variant, this finding should be considered abnormal.

CARTILAGE UNDERCUTTING LABRUM

The base of the acetabular labrum normally has a firm attachment to the bony acetabulum. However, on occasion, intermediate signal intensity can be found on MR imaging at the junction of the articular surface of the labrum and the acetabulum. In their study that correlated MR arthrography with anatomic examination of cadaveric hips, Czerny and colleagues[2] showed that this area of increased signal corresponds to the attachment of the labrum to the acetabular cartilage. This should not be mistaken for a tear if the signal is hypointense to fluid or injected arthrographic contrast material, especially if it has a signal intensity similar to that of the hyaline cartilage and smoothly parallels the labral base and acetabular rim. Furthermore, the adjacent hyaline cartilage surface is usually smooth when the findings are related to cartilage undercutting of the labrum (**Fig. 1**) but may be irregular if there is a true labral tear.

SUBLABRAL SULCUS

There has been much debate in the literature over the existence and location of a normal sublabral sulcus that could be misinterpreted as a labral tear. In a histologic study of fetal acetabula, Walker and Goldsmith[10] described an anterosuperior sublabral sulcus. However, no definite sulcus was identified on the gross hip specimens, suggesting that the sulcus seen on histology may have been related to a tissue-processing artifact. Dinauer and colleagues[9] described a normal posteroinferior sublabral groove in 22.4% of 58 patients on

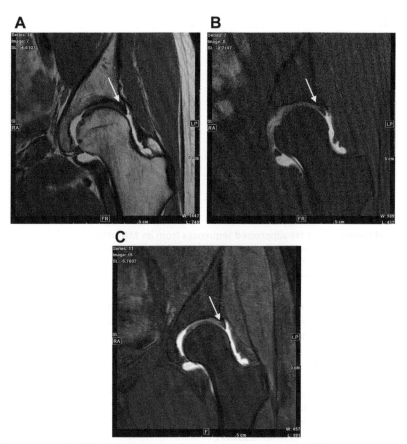

Fig. 1. Coronal proton density (*A*), T1 fat-suppressed (*B*), and T2 fat-suppressed (*C*) sequences show hyaline cartilage interposed between the acetabular rim and the superior acetabular labrum (*arrows*). The cartilage undercutting the labrum is isointense to the rest of the articular cartilage and hypointense to injected contrast material. In addition, the adjacent articular cartilage is normal.

MR arthrography. In a study on 121 hip arthroscopies, Saddik and colleagues[11] found sublabral sulci in 25% of patients, 44% of which were anterosuperior, 48% of which were posteroinferior, 4% of which were anteroinferior, and 4% of which were posterosuperior. Using a clock face to describe the position of labral findings in which the 12 o'clock position was superior and the nine o'clock position was anterior, Studler and colleagues[12] compared the MR arthrography findings in 57 patients to arthroscopic findings and reported 7 sublabral recesses at the 8-o'clock position, 2 at the 9-o'clock position, and 1 at the 10-o'clock position. They found that a sublabral sulcus does not extend through the entire labral base and that sublabral contrast maintained a linear morphology (**Fig. 2**). In their study, sublabral sulci showed no abnormal signal in the labrum adjacent to the sulcus, there were no adjacent cartilage lesions or osseous abnormalities, and there were no ganglion cysts. The depth of the labral tears was greater than that of the sulci, but the 2 entities did not differ in longitudinal extent. They

concluded that arthrographic contrast material extending through the base of the labrum should be considered as an indication of a labral tear.

Other investigators have disputed the existence of a normal sublabral sulcus. Czerny and colleagues[2] found no evidence of a normal sublabral sulcus in their study of MR imaging arthrograms on 40 symptomatic patients and 6 cadaveric hip joint specimens, and Petersilge and colleagues[13] found no evidence of a normal sublabral sulcus in their study of 10 patients who underwent MR arthrography and subsequent arthroscopy. As a result, many investigators have concluded that there likely is a normal sublabral sulcus posteroinferiorly just above the transverse ligament. However, similar findings in the anterior or anterosuperior labrum should be carefully evaluated because many of these defects represent true labral tears.

Often imagers rely on direct arthroscopic visualization to determine whether an MR finding represents a tear or a sulcus. However, it should be remembered that arthroscopy is an imperfect gold

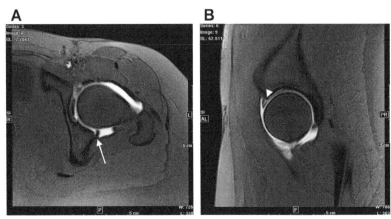

Fig. 2. Axial (*A*) and sagittal (*B*) T1 fat-suppressed sequences from an MR arthrogram examination show injected contrast undercutting the posterior acetabular labrum (*arrow*). This finding was interpreted as a tear but was shown to represent a sublabral foramen on arthroscopy. The patient also had an anterior labral tear that was addressed at arthroscopy (*arrowhead*).

standard because there is no consensus among arthroscopists about what represents the normal labral appearance. Use of higher-resolution MR imaging, such as 3-tesla imaging, frequently reveals a shallow, smooth defect along the articular surface of the superior and anterosuperior labral base, which may represent a sublabral sulcus (**Fig. 3**). These defects generally do not involve more than a third of the labral thickness, and the width of the defect is often larger than its depth. In addition, there should not be any adjacent hyaline cartilage

loss. On arthrography, contrast should smoothly enter these sulci and should not enter the labral substance.

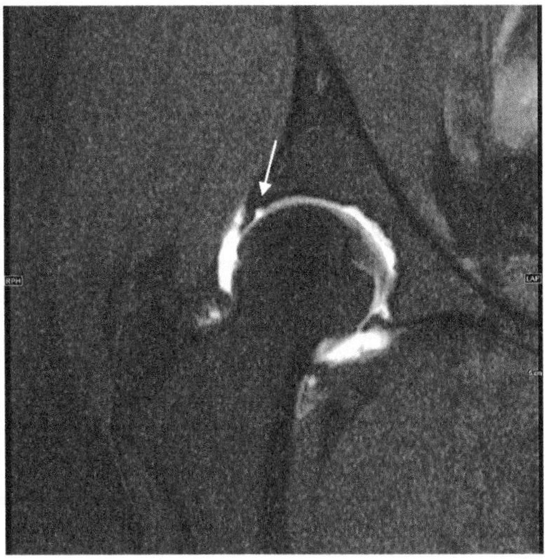

TRANSVERSE LIGAMENT

The acetabulum nearly completely covers the femoral head, with the exception of its anteroinferior aspect, where there is a lack of bone and cartilage. This anteroinferior aspect of the acetabulum is spanned by the transverse acetabular ligament, which, with the acetabular labrum, forms a complete ring around the acetabulum. The transverse ligament attaches to the acetabular rim anteriorly and posteriorly and to the ligamentum teres femoris. Where the transverse ligament meets the acetabular labrum, there occurs a normal cleft that can be mistaken for an acetabular labral tear (**Fig. 4**). Dinauer and colleagues[9] found a cleft at the junction of the transverse ligament and the anterior labrum in 32.8% of hips.

SYNOVIAL HERNIATION PITS

Femoral fibrocystic changes are common anteriorly at the junction of the head and neck, with some investigators reporting an incidence of up to 33% (**Fig. 5**). This finding was first described by Pitt and colleagues[14] in 1982. Although the cause is idiopathic, the investigators speculated that the cysts appeared as a result of repetitive herniation of fluid and synovium related to the overlying joint capsule through small perforations in the cortical bone. More recently, Leunig and colleagues[15] proposed that the fibrocystic changes in the anterior part of the bone were not incidental but related to repetitive impingement of the femoral neck and the anterosuperior

Fig. 3. A coronal T1 fat-suppressed image from an MR arthrogram shows a shallow, smooth defect along the articular surface of the superior labrum (*arrow*) without adjacent hyaline cartilage loss that could represent a sublabral sulcus. Intra-articular local anesthetic was administered during the arthrogram, although the patient's symptoms did not significantly improve during postprocedural provocative maneuvers.

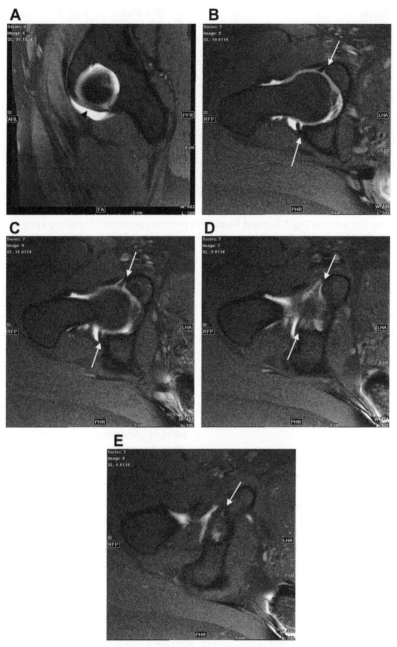

Fig. 4. Sagittal (*A*) and sequential axial T1 fat-suppressed (*B–E*) images through the inferior aspect of the right hip from an MR arthrogram show the transverse ligament along the inferior acetabular margin (*arrowhead*). Contrast undercuts the junction of the transverse ligament and labrum anteriorly and posteriorly (*arrows*).

acetabulum. On radiography, these cysts often appear as lucent lesions in the anterior part of the femoral head/neck junction with a thin peripheral sclerotic rim. They are most commonly small, measuring a few millimeters, but can be larger than a centimeter and may also grow.[16] On MR imaging, the cysts are usually hyperintense to skeletal muscle on T2-weighted sequences and may approach the signal intensity of fluid. Occasionally, there may be marrow edema associated with these cysts, which may manifest as an area of increased radiotracer uptake on bone scintigraphy.[17,18] A defect in the overlying cortical bone may be seen in larger cysts, and there may be

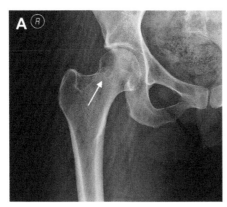
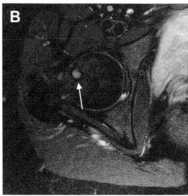

Fig. 5. Anteroposterior radiograph (*A*) and axial T2 fat-suppressed image (*B*) of the right hip show a synovial herniation pit along the anterior right femoral head/neck junction (*arrows*). On radiography, the lesion is radiolucent, with a thin smooth sclerotic rim, whereas on MR imaging, it is T2 hyperintense compared with the adjacent marrow.

other associated findings of femoroacetabular impingement, such as anterosuperior labral tears, acetabular overcoverage leading to pincer impingement, or femoral head asphericity associated with cam-type impingement.[15,19] Thus, synovial herniation pits may suggest alterations in hip biomechanics leading to abnormalities, and proper recognition of this finding may help to direct the patient toward proper treatment.

OS ACETABULI

The origin of bone fragments along the acetabular rim, called os acetabuli or os acetabulare (**Fig. 6**), has long been a topic of debate. First described by Albinus in 1737, these fragments can occur in the process of normal acetabular development in young people aged 6 to 20 years.[20] In a study of 1111 pelvic radiographs, Arho[21] found that 2% to 3% of asymptomatic patients had an os acetabuli.

Some investigators have attributed these acetabuli to nonunion of secondary acetabular ossification centers, incomplete healing of acetabular rim fractures, or ossifications within the acetabular labrum.[22] Ossification of the anterosuperior acetabulum is also found in the setting of cam-type femoroacetabular impingement syndrome, in which abnormal offset at the femoral head/neck junction causes trauma to and premature degeneration and ossification of the acetabular labrum. Acetabular ossification can also occur after trauma, rickets, osteomyelitis, and osteochondritis dissecans.[20]

PERILABRAL RECESS

The hip joint capsule attaches directly to the osseous rim of the acetabulum, supported by the ischiofemoral ligament posteriorly and the iliofemoral and pubofemoral ligaments anteriorly. The

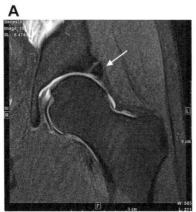
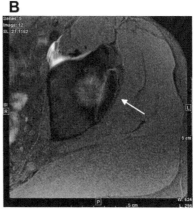

Fig. 6. Coronal (*A*) and axial (*B*) T1 fat-suppressed sequences from an MR arthrogram of the left hip show a large os acetabuli (*arrows*) in a characteristic superolateral position along the actebular rim.

distal capsule inserts at the base of the femoral neck (**Fig. 7**). A normal sulcus exists between the medial joint capsule and the acetabular labrum. In the anterior and posterior aspects of the acetabulum, the capsule attaches directly at the base of the labrum. Superiorly, the capsule attaches several millimeters above the labrum. Thus, the perilabral recess is larger superiorly than anteriorly and posteriorly. The perilabral recess is a potential space not always appreciated on nonarthrographic examinations. On routine nonarthrographic hip MR imaging, joint fluid trapped within the perilabral recess can mimic a paralabral cyst and erroneously suggest an adjacent labral tear. Joint distension by arthrographic contrast material provides better visualization of this recess and may help distinguish between joint fluid and perilabral cyst.[6,13,23]

SUPRA-ACETABULAR FOSSA AND STELLATE LESION

The supra-acetabular fossa is an additional cavity in the superior, weight-bearing region of the acetabulum seen at the 12-o'clock position and is frequently filled with fibrous tissue. It is usually easily distinguishable from an osteochondral lesion because it has relatively smooth margins and there is normal underlying marrow signal (**Fig. 8**).

The stellate lesion (also called the stellate crease) is another anatomic variant separate

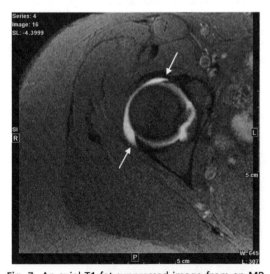

Fig. 7. An axial T1 fat-suppressed image from an MR arthrogram of the right hip shows normal anterior and posterior perilabral recesses (*arrows*). Injected intra-articular contrast aids visualization of these normal recesses by distending the joint capsule and separating the capsule from the labrum.

from and medial to the supra-acetabular fossa. The stellate lesion represents a bare area within the acetabular articular surface above the anterosuperior margin of the acetabulum (**Fig. 9**). It is more commonly found in young adults but can also be seen in older people. On MR imaging, the lesion can appear irregular and could be mistaken for an osteochondral lesion or chondromalacia. On arthroscopy, the stellate lesion appears as a linear indentation in the acetabular roof, where the cartilage is focally discontinuous, and there may be a subchondral osseous fragment attached to the acetabular fossa by a hypointense plica. The stellate lesion is also separate from the triradiate cartilage, which represents the developmental remnant of the triradiate cartilage. The physeal scar is found in the medial aspect of the acetabulum, and it is important not to mistake the triradiate cartilage for a stellate lesion or fracture.[24,25]

ILIOPSOAS BURSA

The iliopsoas bursa is the largest bursa about the hip, located subjacent to the iliopsoas myotendinous junction, anterior to the hip joint capsule, and lateral to the femoral vessels.[26] A normal iliopsoas bursa may be collapsed and not visible on MR imaging, although distention with a small amount of fluid can also be seen in asymptomatic hips. In MR arthrography, intra-articular contrast material can be seen within the bursa because it communicates with the hip joint in 15% of people (**Fig. 10**). Contrast extending into the iliopsoas bursa does not necessarily indicate capsular disruption because such a communication can be either congenital or acquired. In instances of acquired communication, chronic friction from the iliopsoas tendon on the joint capsule causes synovitis and ultimately tearing of the capsule that allows joint fluid to escape into and distend the bursa.[27] Iliopsoas bursitis can be caused by osteoarthritis, rheumatoid arthritis, gout, osteonecrosis, hip arthroplasty, and other conditions.[27] A distended iliopsoas bursa often subtends a horseshoe configuration, with 2 lobes extending anteriorly on either side of the iliopsoas tendon. A distended bursa may extend cranially into the pelvis along the iliopsoas muscle.[26]

ACCESSORY ILIACUS TENDON

Iliopsoas tendon abnormality is an occasional cause of anterior hip or groin pain that may radiate distally or produce a "snap" sensation. As in the pathology of other tendons, MR findings of iliopsoas tendinopathy include tendon thickening,

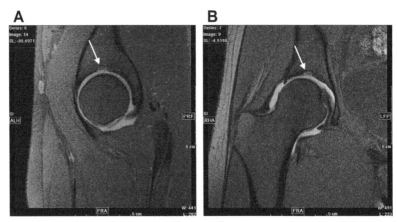

Fig. 8. Sagittal (*A*) and coronal (*B*) T1 fat-suppressed images from an MR arthrogram of the right hip in a 15-year-old patient demonstrate a focal indentation in the superior acetabulum at the 12-o'clock position (*arrows*). Arthroscopy confirmed a superior labral tear with adjacent cartilage irregularity (not shown); however, the cartilage abnormality did not extend medially to involve the area of this finding.

intermediate intrasubstance signal abnormalities, and partial or complete tears. Tendon abnormality is frequently associated with iliopsoas bursitis. The accessory iliacus tendon is a common variant, seen in 66% of MR arthrograms, which can mimic iliopsoas tendon pathology.[28] Although this variant is not usually symptomatic, one anatomic study on 68 cadavers found 3 instances in which the accessory slip pierced the femoral nerve. The investigators speculated that this finding could potentially lead to nerve impingement.[29] On non–fat-suppressed sequences, there may be a small tendon paralleling the iliopsoas major tendon separated by a fat plane that can simulate a longitudinal tendon tear. In these cases, frequency selective or short-tau inversion recovery fat-suppressed sequences may be useful to distinguish between a tendon tear and an anatomic variation (**Fig. 11**).[30]

TUBULAR TRACKING OF CONTRAST IN ARTHROGRAPHY

In 2006, Lien and colleagues[31] described intraosseous tracking of contrast material in computed tomography and MR arthrography of the hip. The tracks are linear, blind-ending structures that originate from the acetabular fossa at or close to its margin with the acetabular cartilage (**Fig. 12**). The track orifices measured 0.6 to 1.5 mm (mean, 1.2 mm), and the track length was 0.4 to 1.7 cm (mean, 1.1 cm). Tubular acetabular intraosseous contrast tracking was seen in 23 (16%) of 145 hips examined and in 19 (15%) of 123 symptomatic hips. Because incidence was nearly equal in symptomatic and asymptomatic populations, this finding is thought to be an unlikely source of hip pain.

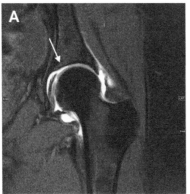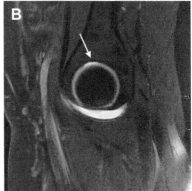

Fig. 9. Coronal (*A*) and sagittal (*B*) T1 fat-suppressed images from an MR arthrogram of the left hip in a 23-year-old patient depict near full-thickness absence of the acetabular articular cartilage medial to the 12-o'clock position without underlying marrow signal abnormalities consistent with a stellate lesion (*arrows*).

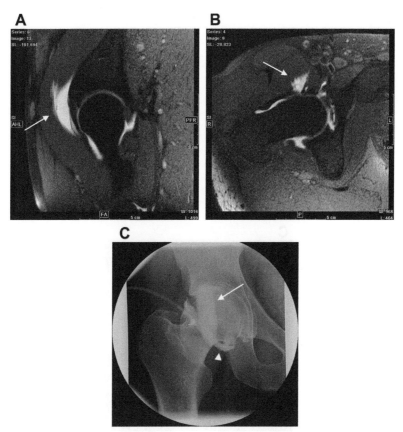

Fig. 10. Sagittal (*A*) and axial (*B*) T1 fat-suppressed images from a right hip MR arthrogram show a horseshoe-shaped contrast collection deep to the iliopsoas tendon and extending from the hip joint along either side of the iliopsoas tendon, which represents a normal iliopsoas bursa (*arrows*). The bursa extends cranially along the iliacus muscle. An anteroposterior fluoroscopic image (*C*) from this patient's arthrography shows injected contrast surrounding the base of the femoral head (*arrowhead*) as well as extending into the iliopsoas bursa (*arrow*). Both the MR and fluoroscopic images show communication of the hip joint and bursa, with contrast tracking cranially along the iliopsoas muscle.

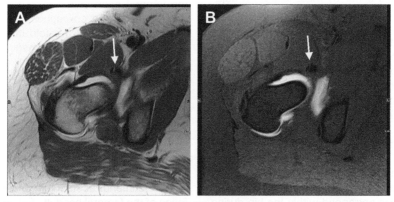

Fig. 11. An axial proton density image from a right hip MR arthrogram (*A*) shows increased signal in the iliopsoas tendon (*arrow*) that may simulate a longitudinal tear. However, this structure loses signal intensity (*arrow*) on the corresponding T1 fat-suppressed image (*B*). This finding represents fat between the iliopsoas and accessory iliacus tendons rather than a longitudinal tear.

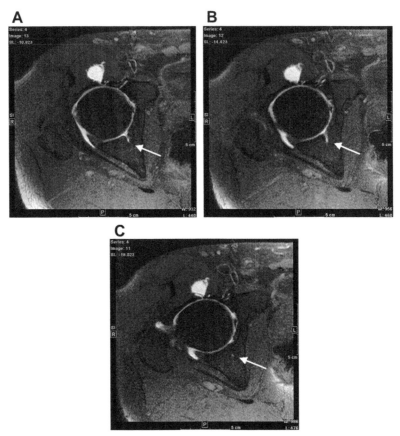

Fig. 12. Sequential axial T1 fat-suppressed images from a right hip MR arthrogram (*A–C*) show tracking of injected contrast into a blind-ending tubular structure from the posteromedial acetabulum to the ischium (*arrows*).

PLICAE AND THE PECTINOFOVEAL FOLD

Plicae are embryologic remnants that are occasionally seen in synovial joints as areas of capsular or synovial folds that may encroach on the joint space. They are generally asymptomatic but may cause symptoms either by mass effect on adjacent structures or by impingement between 2 structures. Plicae are frequent in the knee, although symptomatic plicae have been described in other joints such as the elbow or tibiotalar joints. Symptomatic plicae in the hip are uncommon, with only 4 published case reports.[32–34] However, when they occur they may produce progressive pain with activity, an audible click and possibly crepitus, or effusion. Fu and colleagues[35] described 3 locations: labral, ligamentous, and neck plicae. Of these, the labral plica is most likely to be symptomatic because it is located parallel to either the acetabular labrum or the transverse ligament and can be entrapped within the hip during movement. The ligamentous variety is located within the acetabular fossa, whereas the neck variety is near the capsular reflection around the

femoral neck. Both of these are unlikely to be entrapped and therefore unlikely to be symptomatic.

On the other hand, the pectinofoveal fold is a common anatomic variant seen on MR arthrography as a linear band paralleling the inferior margin of the femoral neck that may attach to the femoral neck or the joint capsule (**Fig. 13**). Blankenbaker and colleagues[36] recently showed that the incidence of this fold in a series of 152 patients was 95% on MR imaging and 99% in arthroscopy. The fold itself is unlikely to be symptomatic and has little clinical significance. However, this finding should not be mistaken for a plica, which can potentially be symptomatic.

LIGAMENTUM TERES

The ligamentum teres is a fibrovascular structure that primarily arises from the transverse ligament along the inferior acetabulum and inserts into the fovea of the femoral head. Its function, particularly in adults, has been widely debated, although some investigators think that it may provide stability to the hip, particularly in adduction, flexion, and

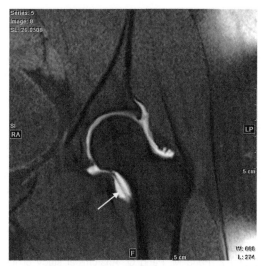

Fig. 13. Coronal T1 fat-suppressed image from a left hip MR arthrogram shows a linear hypointense structure paralleling the inferior margin of the femoral neck that represents a pectinofoveal fold (*arrow*).

external rotation. In addition, it contains nerve endings that may provide improved hip proprioception.[37,38] On MR imaging, the ligamentum teres is normally a single, flat, thin structure with low signal intensity on all pulse sequences that may become more oval or bilobed at its foveal attachment.[39] Demange and colleagues[40] have suggested that the ligamentum teres consists of 3 bundles. Although these bundles are generally indistinguishable from one another, a recent study by Sadej and colleagues[41] involving 102 MR arthrograms with high-resolution MR imaging demonstrated 2 or 3 separate bundles in 11% of their MR studies. However, it may be difficult to routinely distinguish between bifid or trifid ligamentum teres and longitudinal teres on MR imaging. Finally, some patients, particularly those with developmental hip dysplasia, may have congenital absence of the ligamentum teres,[42] and absence of the ligamentum teres in these patients should not be construed as a chronic tear.

SUMMARY

Several variants in the morphology and imaging appearance of the hip have been described, which may imitate pathologic conditions or may alter the biomechanics of the hip to produce abnormalities. It is important for imagers and clinicians to be aware of these variations and potential pitfalls to prevent erroneous diagnosis. In some instances, it may be necessary to perform MR arthrography with concomitant intra-articular local anesthetic injection to help distinguish between developmental variants and symptomatic pathologic states whenever there are equivocal findings.

REFERENCES

1. Blankenbaker DG, De Smet AA, Keene JS, et al. Classification and localization of acetabular labral tears. Skeletal Radiol 2007;36:391–7.
2. Czerny C, Hofmann S, Urban M, et al. MR arthrography of the adult acetabular capsular-labral complex: correlation with surgery and anatomy. AJR Am J Roentgenol 1999;173(2):345–9.
3. Magee T, Hinson G. Association of paralabral cysts with acetabular disorders. AJR Am J Roentgenol 2000;174(5):1381–4.
4. Hodler J, Yu JS, Goodwin D, et al. MR arthrography of the hip: improved imaging of the acetabular labrum with histologic correlation in cadavers. AJR Am J Roentgenol 1995;165:887–91.
5. Cotten A, Boutry N, Demondion X, et al. Acetabular labrum: MRI in asymptomatic volunteers. J Comput Assist Tomogr 1998;22:1–7.
6. Petersilge CA. Chronic adult hip pain: MR arthrography of the hip. Radiographics 2000;20:S43–52.
7. Lecouvet FE, Vande Berg BC, Malghem J, et al. MR imaging of the acetabular labrum: variations in 200 asymptomatic hips. AJR Am J Roentgenol 1996; 167:1025–8.
8. Tirman PFJ, Feller JF, Palmer WE, et al. The Buford complex—a variation of normal shoulder anatomy: MR arthrographic imaging features. AJR Am J Roentgenol 1996;166:869–72.
9. Dinauer PA, Murphy KP, Carroll JF. Sublabral sulcus at the posteroinferior acetabulum: a potential pitfall in MR arthrography diagnosis of acetabular labral tears. AJR Am J Roentgenol 2004;183:1745–53.
10. Walker JM, Goldsmith CH. Morphometric study of the fetal development of the human hip joint: significance for congenital hip disease. Yale J Biol Med 1981;54(6):411–37.
11. Saddik D, Troupis J, Tirman P, et al. Prevalence and location of acetabular sublabral sulci at hip arthroscopy with retrospective MRI review. AJR Am J Roentgenol 2006;187(5):W507–11.
12. Studler U, Kalberer F, Leunig M, et al. MR arthrography of the hip: differentiation between an anterior sublabral recess as a normal variant and a labral tear. Radiology 2008;249:947–54.
13. Petersilge CA, Haque MA, Petersilge WJ, et al. Acetabular labral tears: evaluation with MR arthrography. Radiology 1996;200:231–5.
14. Pitt MJ, Graham AR, Shipman JH, et al. Herniation pit of the femoral neck. AJR Am J Roentgenol 1982;138(6):1115–21.
15. Leunig M, Beck M, Kalhor M, et al. Fibrocystic changes at anterosuperior femoral neck: prevalence

in hips with femoroacetabular impingement. Radiology 2005;236(1):237–46.

16. Crabbe JP, Martel W, Matthews LS. Rapid growth of femoral herniation pit. AJR Am J Roentgenol 1992; 159(5):1038–40.

17. Swayne LC, Colston WC. Scintigraphic findings of a femoral neck herniation pit. Clin Nucl Med 1996; 21(3):258.

18. Sopov V, Fuchs D, Bar-Meir E, et al. Clinical spectrum of asymptomatic femoral neck abnormal uptake on bone scintigraphy. J Nucl Med 2002;43(4):484–6.

19. Beall DP, Sweet CF, Martin HD, et al. Imaging findings of femoroacetabular impingement syndrome. Skeletal Radiol 2005;34(11):691–701.

20. Klaue K, Durnin CW, Ganz R. The acetabular rim syndrome. J Bone Joint Surg Br 1991;73(3):423–9.

21. Arho AO. Accessory bones of extremities in roentgen picture. Duodecim 1940;56:399–410.

22. Hergan K, Oser W, Moriggl B. Acetabular ossicles: normal variant or disease entity? Eur Radiol 2000; 10(4):624–8.

23. Chatha DS, Arora R. MR imaging of the normal hip. Magn Reson Imaging Clin N Am 2005;13(4): 605–15.

24. Villar R. Arthroscopic anatomy of the hip. In: Byrd JWT, editor. Operative hip arthroscopy. 2nd edition. New York: Springer-Verlag; 2005. p. 117–28.

25. Stoller DW, editor. Magnetic resonance imaging in orthopaedics and sports medicine. 3rd edition. Philadelphia: Lippincott, Williams and Wilkins; 2006.

26. Varma DG, Richli WR, Charnsangavej C, et al. MR appearance of the distended iliopsoas bursa. AJR Am J Roentgenol 1991;156:1025–8.

27. Bianchi S, Martinoli C, Keller A, et al. Giant iliopsoas bursitis: sonographic findings with magnetic resonance correlations. J Clin Ultrasound 2002;30:437–41.

28. Tatu L, Parratte B, Vuillier F, et al. Descriptive anatomy of the femoral portion of the iliopsoas muscle. Anatomical basis of anterior snapping of the hip. Surg Radiol Anat 2001;23(6):371–4.

29. Spratt JD, Logan BM, Abrahams PH. Variant slips of psoas and iliacus muscles, with splitting of the femoral nerve. Clin Anat 1996;9(6):401–4.

30. Polster JM, Elgabaly M, Lee H, et al. Normal anatomy leading to misdiagnosis of the iliopsoas

tendon pathology. Society of Skeletal Radiology 13th Annual Meeting. Orlando (FL). March 18–21, 2007.

31. Lien L, Hunter J, Chan Y. Tubular acetabular intraosseous contrast tracking in MR arthrography of the hip: prevalence, clinical significance, and mechanisms of development. AJR Am J Roentgenol 2006; 187:807–10.

32. Frich LH, Lauritzen J, Juhl M. Arthroscopy in diagnosis and treatment of hip disorders. Orthopedics 1989;12:389–92.

33. Hélénon CH, Bergevin H, Aubert JD, et al. Plication of hip synovia at upper border femoral neck. J Radiol 1986;67:737–40.

34. Atlihan D, Jones DC, Guanche CA. Arthroscopic treatment of a symptomatic hip plica. Clin Orthop Relat Res 2003;411:174–7.

35. Fu Z, Peng M, Peng Q. Anatomical study of the synovial plicae of the hip joint. Clin Anat 1997; 10(4):235–8.

36. Blankenbaker DG, Davis KW, De Smet AA, et al. MRI appearance of the pectinofoveal fold. AJR Am J Roentgenol 2009;192(1):93–5.

37. Rao J, Zhou YX, Villar RN. Injury to the ligamentum teres. Mechanism, findings, and results of treatment. Clin Sports Med 2001;20(4):791–9, vii.

38. Byrd JW, Jones KS. Traumatic rupture of the ligamentum teres as a source of hip pain. Arthroscopy 2004;20(4):385–91.

39. Armfield DR, Towers JD, Robertson DD. Radiographic and MR imaging of the athletic hip. Clin Sports Med 2006;25(2):211–39, viii.

40. Demange MK, Kakuda CMS, Pereira CAM, et al. Influence of the femoral head ligament on hip mechanical function. Acta Orthop Bras 2007;15: 187–90.

41. Sadej P, Zoga A, Morrison W. MR arthrographic appearance of ligamentum teres tears: variations of normal and patterns of injury. American Roentgen Ray Society 2010 Annual Meeting. San Diego (CA). March 2–7, 2010.

42. Ipplito E, Ishii Y, Ponseti IV. Histologic, histochemical and ultrastructural studies of the hip joint capsule and ligamentum teres in congenital dislocation of the hip. Clin Orthop 1980;146:246–58.

Magnetic Resonance Imaging Pitfalls and Normal Variations: The Knee

Thomas Slattery, MD*, Nancy Major, MD

KEYWORDS
- MR imaging • Knee • Pitfalls • Tears

With its excellent soft tissue contrast capabilities and ease of acquisition of multiple imaging planes, magnetic resonance (MR) imaging has become the standard for definitive evaluation of the knee across the spectrum of pathologic conditions. The technique has excellent ability to evaluate the bone, cartilage, ligaments, and tendons in a single examination. In short, it is highly accurate with sensitivity and specificity of up to 90% to 95% for the menisci and nearly 100% for the cruciate ligaments. Like all joints imaged with MR imaging, the knee has many potential pitfalls and anatomic variations. The interpreting radiologist must be well versed in this knowledge to avoid reporting pathologic conditions when it is not present and to not misinterpret subtle diagnoses for normal variation and thus deprive a patient of a timely path toward appropriate treatment. In this article, multiple examples of variations and potential pitfalls are provided along with examples of knee internal derangements at MR imaging, which contrast the mimics. Also included are several examples of pathologic conditions that may clinically mimic more serious lesions, and if these conditions are not characterized properly, then the pitfall of potentially unnecessary invasive treatments could ensue.

MR IMAGING OF THE KNEE: TECHNICAL CONSIDERATIONS AND PULSE SEQUENCES

A dedicated knee coil is recommended for optimal knee imaging. There are multiple products in use with similar results. Such coils are of considerate expense in the tens of thousands of dollars but are vital for optimal results. A small field of view is ideal in the range of 14 to 16 cm depending on patient size. Most centers use a 4-mm slice thickness with a range of 3 to 5 mm being most often used. A 0.4-mm interslice gap reduces cross talk but is not needed if volume imaging is used. Typical matrices used for the knee are 256 × 192 or 256 × 256. Positioning the patient with the knee at rest is usually at about 5° of external rotation. This position optimizes the evaluation of the anterior cruciate ligament (ACL), placing it in the plane of sagittal imaging. When selecting pulse sequences, it is an important consideration to have a sequence with a short echo time (TE) to best evaluate for meniscal tears and the posterior cruciate ligament (PCL). This evaluation may be done with conventional spin echo T1-weighted (T1W), proton density (PD), or gradient echo sequences. For meniscal imaging, a sagittal PD sequence with fat suppression is advised. The fat suppression provides better aesthetic evaluation of the menisci (much like meniscal windows did). For evaluation of the cruciate ligaments, cartilage, and bones, a T2-weighted (T2W) sequence with fat suppression is recommended. A gradient echo imaging is adequate for the evaluation of cartilage and ligaments but is suboptimal for the evaluation of pathologic conditions of bone marrow, and thus another marrow-sensitive sequence is needed. The coronal plane is useful for the examination of

Department of Radiology, Hospital of the University of Pennsylvania, 399 South 34th Street, Penn Tower Suite 100, Philadelphia, PA 19104, USA
* Corresponding author.
E-mail address: Thomas.slattery@uphs.upenn.edu

Magn Reson Imaging Clin N Am 18 (2010) 675–689
doi:10.1016/j.mric.2010.09.004

the collateral ligaments and cartilage and also gives a second evaluation of the cruciate ligaments when the sagittal plane is not conclusive. Fat-suppressed T2W imaging is especially useful for ligaments, cartilage, and bone marrow. In addition, the identification of meniscocapsular separation is made easier with this technique. Fluid noted between the medial meniscus and medial collateral ligament (MCL) is diagnostic of a meniscocapsular separation. A normal small fat pad in this region may get misconstrued as fluid if fat suppression is not used. T1W imaging in the coronal plane was often used yet added no advantage over T2W imaging and has been largely replaced with T2W imaging. In the axial plane, evaluation of the patellar cartilage, trochlear cartilage, and medial patellar plicae can readily be performed. There is also a second or third look at the cruciate ligaments and a second look at the collateral ligaments. MR arthrography has had some utility in the differentiation of postoperative changes versus a new meniscal tear, but this discussion is beyond the scope of this article.

MENISCI

The menisci are C-shaped, fibrocartilaginous structures and are thicker at their periphery than at their center. The menisci are made of thick collagen fibers mostly arranged circumferentially, with radial fibers extending from the capsule, between the circumferential fibers. The superior surfaces of the menisci are concave and the inferior surfaces are flat, which facilitates congruent relationships of the femur and tibia.[1] The posterior horn of the medial meniscus is larger than the anterior horn. In the lateral meniscus, the anterior and posterior horns are equal in size. It is an abnormal finding if the posterior horn of a meniscus is smaller than the anterior horn. In adults, a normal meniscus is low in signal. In children and adolescents, there is intermediate to high signal in the posterior horns near their attachment to the capsule, related to normal vascularity (**Fig. 1**). Because of the vascularity at the periphery of the menisci, tears in this region may be repaired. However, at the center, where there is minimal vascularity, most of these tears cannot be repaired.

Abnormal signal detected within a meniscus, which does not abut the articular surface indicates intrasubstance or myxoid degeneration (**Fig. 2**). This degeneration may be related to wear and tear with aging, but this relation is not entirely certain. This degeneration is inconsequential in that it is asymptomatic and does not correlate with risk of tears. The important consideration is

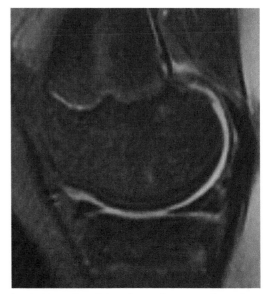

Fig. 1. Normal peripheral vascular zone of meniscus. Sagittal PD-weighted image with fat suppression shows globular high signal within the posterior horn of the medial meniscus in an adolescent, reflecting normal vascularity, which can be confused with a tear.

to differentiate it from meniscal cysts, which may be symptomatic and are discussed later.

High signal that can clearly be seen to disrupt an articular surface of the meniscus is diagnostic of

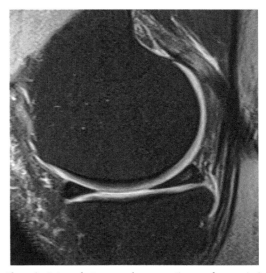

Fig. 2. Intrasubstance degeneration of menisci. Sagittal PD-weighted image with fat suppression showing globular increased signal within the posterior horn of the medial meniscus not abutting the articular surface. This finding is common particularly in older patients and at times may pose a challenge to differentiate from tear when the signal approaches the meniscal surface.

a tear. Signal not disrupting the surface, as mentioned earlier, indicates degeneration. In about 10% of cases, the disruption of the articular surface is not always clearly identified.[2,3] In these cases, the site of the questionable finding should be reported for the treating surgeon to correlate with their clinical examination and, if needed, arthroscopy.

Many patterns of meniscal tears have been described. A brief review of the imaging findings of the tears is provided to contrast the multiple mimics of tears described later. Important features describing tears include the site in the meniscus, extent of tear, and associated findings, such as meniscal cysts. Most common is the oblique or horizontal tear (synonyms) of the undersurface of the posterior horn of the medial meniscus, believed to most commonly be degenerative and not related to trauma (**Fig. 3**). Vertical longitudinal tears or bucket-handle tears make up about 10% of tears. These tears can be detected when the normal two consecutive slabs of rectangular meniscal tissue are not seen through the body of a meniscus. The absent second slab of meniscal tissue is because of the displaced portion of the meniscus. Recognizing the absence of the body has sensitivities for bucket-handle tears in the range of 71% to 97%.[4,5] The displaced fragment is most often found in the intercondylar notch. The fragment could also be found to lie in front of the PCL, which is called the double PCL sign (**Fig. 4**). If flipped over the anterior horn, this displaced fragment may be called an anterior flipped meniscus sign.

Another cause of absence of body segments is the radial or free edge tear (**Fig. 5**). These are frequent tears and can have an incidence as high as 15%.[6] These types of tears may be asymptomatic. Three variations of the appearance may be encountered, the ghost, cleft, and truncated triangle. The ghost meniscus is seen when the tear completely traverses the meniscus. An MR imaging slice parallel to the tear shows partial volume averaging of the surrounding tissues, leading to a gray signal. This tear reduces the spring resistance (hoop strength) of the meniscus and may lead to extrusion of the meniscus and accelerated osteoarthritis. A cleft appearance to a radial tear is seen when the MR image is perpendicular to the tear. When parallel to the tear, the image shows the truncated triangle appearance.

A tear of the medial meniscus with particular importance for both the radiologist and arthroscopist is the medial flipped meniscus tear (**Fig. 6**). This tear is of high importance for the interpreting radiologist because it may be overlooked at arthroscopy. The flap may flip into the medial gutter beneath the meniscus and should be scrutinized for when the body segments appear thinned or have an inferior defect. The flipped fragment may be well seen on coronal images just inferomedial to the medial meniscus. This flip is yet another cause of the absent body segment on sagittal imaging.[7]

Some deviations from the usual expectation of the 2 body segments of the menisci on sagittal images should be remembered to avoid overinterpretation of pathologic conditions. Smaller patients and children have smaller menisci and may not have 2 body segments visualized. Postsurgical debridement is another cause. Few body segments can also be encountered in examinations of patients with severe osteoarthritis, in

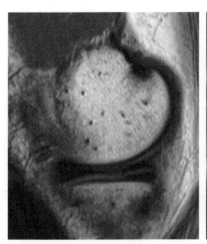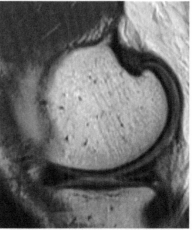

Fig. 3. Horizontal or oblique tear of meniscus. Successive sagittal PD-weighted images show linear high signal extending to the inferior articular surface of the posterior horn of the medial meniscus consistent with an oblique tear, the most common type of meniscal tear.

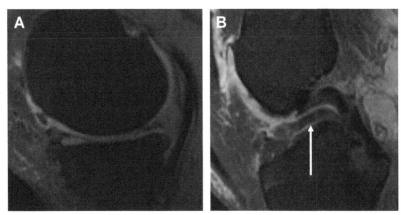

Fig. 4. Bucket-handle tear of meniscus with double PCL sign. Sagittal PD-weighted images with fat suppression shows (A) a markedly deficient body of the medial meniscus and (B) the "handle of the bucket" flipped into the intercondylar notch, the so-called double PCL sign (arrow). The normal PCL is posterosuperior to the flipped fragment. When the body segments of the meniscus are abnormal, a search for the flipped fragment is vital.

which the free edge of the meniscus can be thinned or worn. The lack of identifying displaced meniscal tissue helps with recognizing these pitfalls. The ratio of body segments to anterior and posterior horns (1:2–1:3) is more helpful than absolute numbers.

Meniscal tears have been shown to be more commonly overlooked in the presence of ACL tears. This ignorance occurs because the tears often encountered in this setting are unusual, that is, the tears are often located in the periphery of the medial or lateral menisci and in the posterior horn of the lateral meniscus. Thus, these areas should be closely inspected when the more dramatic finding of ACL tear is encountered.[8]

Additional pathologic conditions important to recognize are the presence of a meniscal cyst and whether or not the cyst is associated with a tear of the meniscus (Fig. 7). The articular surface is not always disrupted when an intra- or parameniscal cyst is present. In an intrameniscal cyst, the signal is expected to be higher than that of intrasubstance degeneration, but overlap may exist. Components of cysts extending beyond the meniscus, or parameniscal cysts, are often of higher T2W signal than those confined within. A diagnosis of intrameniscal cyst is made when the meniscus is swollen in appearance by mass effect from within the meniscus. Describing the location can aid the arthroscopist to closely evaluate the meniscus during surgery. A parameniscal cyst

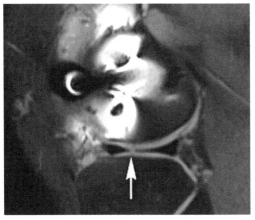

Fig. 5. Radial tear of meniscus. Sagittal T2W image with fat suppression showing a cleft (arrow) in the body of the lateral meniscus consistent with a radial meniscal tear.

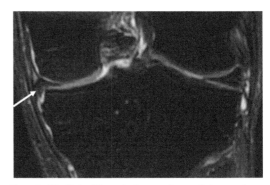

Fig. 6. Medial flipped tear of medial meniscus. Coronal T2W image with fat suppression shows a fragment of the undersurface of the medial meniscus (arrow) displaced inferomedially; an important tear to recognize at MR imaging because it may be occult on routine arthroscopic evaluation.

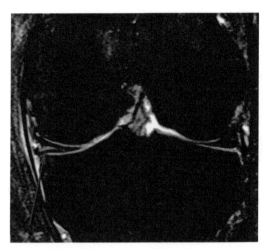

Fig. 7. Intrameniscal and parameniscal cysts. Coronal PD-weighted image with fat suppression shows high signal in a medial meniscus (*long arrow*), which is higher than expected for intrasubstance degeneration. Adjacent medially is a small parameniscal cyst (*short arrow*). Carefully inspect the articular surface for tear when these findings are present. Note that the signal within the intramensical cyst is not fluid signal but that within the paramensical cyst is, which is a common finding.

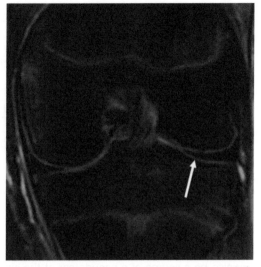

Fig. 8. Discoid meniscus. Coronal T2W image with fat suppression shows prominent medial extension of the lateral meniscus (*arrow*). When scrolling in the sagittal plane, more than 2 of the normal body segments are seen, which is a discoid meniscus; in this case, the meniscus is without tear.

without a tear may not require debridement. Thus, it is important to recognize the presence or absence of a tear.

A discoid meniscus is a congenital malformation of the meniscus, which when severe leads to a disk rather than a C-shape of the meniscus (**Fig. 8**). The diagnosis is suspected when more than 2 body segments are encountered on sagittal images. The lateral meniscus is more frequently associated with a possible incidence of 3%. The medial meniscus is rarely involved. Discoid menisci are prone to cystic degeneration and eventual tears. Even without tears, these menisci may be symptomatic. One such case is the Wrisberg variant of a discoid lateral meniscus. This variant shows a lack of the usual capsular attachments and struts and lacks the normal ligamentous attachment of the posterior horn to the tibia. The only connection is the Wrisberg ligament to the posterior horn. If recognized at surgery, the meniscus can be reattached to the capsule rather than excised potentially, sparing early osteoarthritis. Thus, close inspection of the normal ligamentous and capsular struts is important when analyzing all discoid menisci.[9]

Several special pitfalls of imaging, which mimic meniscal tears, are critical to recognize for accurate interpretation.[10] The transverse ligament runs across the anterior aspect of the knee between the anterior horns of the medial and lateral menisci.

If not followed on subsequent images, the ligament may be mistaken for a meniscal tear near its insertion to the menisci (**Fig. 9**). Another mimicker of tear of the anterior horn is seen in the lateral meniscus as a result of ACL insertion. The anterior horn of the lateral meniscus may have a speckled appearance in up to 60% of cases, a normal variation that could be mistaken for a macerated or torn

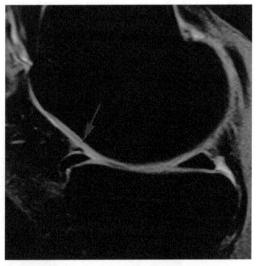

Fig. 9. Normal transverse ligament. Sagittal PD image with fat suppression shows a small structure coursing near the anterior horn of a medial meniscus (*arrow*). When in close approximation to the meniscus, a tear could be mimicked.

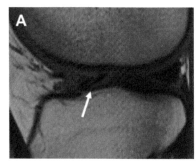 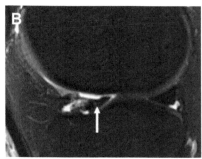

Fig. 10. Speckled anterior horn of lateral meniscus. Sagittal PD-weighted image (*A*) and T2-weighted sagittal image with fat suppression (*B*) show a normal variation of striated or speckled increased signal in the anterior horn of the lateral meniscus near its insertion (*arrows*), not to be confused with a tear.

meniscus (**Fig. 10**). The meniscofemoral ligaments may also be a source of a pseudotear at the site where they insert into the posterior horn of the lateral meniscus. These include the anteriorly situated (relative to the PCL) ligament of Humphrey or posteriorly situated ligament of Wrisberg (**Fig. 11**). Care must be taken to follow these normal structures on subsequent images from the lateral meniscus to the PCL, one or both of these ligaments may be present normally. Pulsation artifact from the popliteal artery could be a source of artifactual meniscal tear, but with routine swapping of phase and frequency, directions to make pulsation extend superior to inferior instead of anterior to posterior should ameliorate this possible error. The magic angle phenomenon can be another source of error, which occurs when a diffuse intermediate signal on PD or T1W images appears when

a structure slopes upward at about 55°, such as in the posterior horn of the lateral meniscus. This signal is not present on longer TE sequences, thus correlation of the T1W or PD images with a T2W sequence should clarify these cases. The popliteus tendon courses between the joint capsule and the posterior horn of the lateral meniscus as it courses obliquely behind the knee. Where it passes the meniscus, a pseudotear appearance could arise or, alternatively, if not discovering its actual location, a vertical tear of the posterior horn of the lateral meniscus could be misinterpreted as a normal structure. Thus, recognition of the expected anatomy and following the course of the structure is vital.

Chondrocalcinosis can be detected on radiographs as a visible calcification in the cartilage of a joint. This condition can commonly occur in the

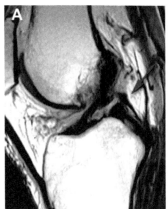 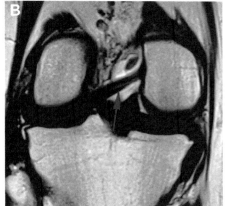

Fig. 11. Meniscofemoral ligament, normal variation. Sagittal PD-weighted (*A*) and coronal PD-weighted image (*B*) show the ligament of Wrisberg (meniscofemoral ligament) coursing posterior to the PCL and then inserting on the posterior horn of the lateral meniscus (*arrows*). Images near the insertion could mimic tear. Knowledge of this anatomy is important to avoid this error.

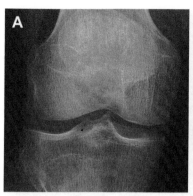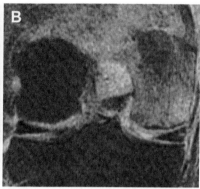

Fig. 12. Chondrocalcinosis. Frontal radiograph (A) and coronal PD-weighted image with fat suppression (B) in the same patient show the value of radiographic correlation. The calcium pyrophosphate deposited within the menisci may show increased or decreased signal on PD images and may mimic tear or obscure true tears. Coincidental bony edema is present in the medial femoral condyle on the MR image related to trauma.

fibrocartilage of a meniscus. It can occur from calcium pyrophosphate dihydrate crystal deposition in pseudogout, which is also known as calcium pyrophosphate dihydrate deposition disease. On T1W and PD images, this calcification may cause increased signal, which could either falsely mimic a meniscal tear or, alternatively, the signal may obscure an actual tear leading to a false negative. Correlation with clinical history as always with sound radiographic correlation helps avoid this pitfall (Fig. 12).[11]

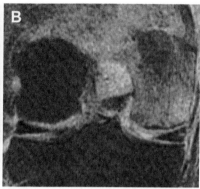

Fig. 13. Meniscal flounce. Sagittal PD image shows a wavy appearance of the medial meniscus, referred to as flounce, which is thought to be related to ligamentous laxity and in and of itself not thought to be clinically significant.

Yet another potential pitfall is meniscal flounce (Fig. 13), a wavy or folded appearance of the inner edge of the medial meniscus. This appearance is believed to be a normal finding, possibly associated with ligamentous laxity but not necessarily indicative of a ligamentous tear. An incidence of 0.2% has been reported. The meniscus takes on a wrinkled appearance from buckling of the inner edge. Flounce is not believed to be clinically significant.[11]

LIGAMENTS

MR imaging is highly accurate for tears of the ACL. Accuracy approaches 95% to 100%.[12] The normal ACL runs parallel to the roof of the intercondylar notch and often has a striated appearance with internal high signal. It is well imaged with T2W sagittal images, with axial or coronal images occasionally aiding in inconclusive cases. A tear is generally obvious with an explosive appearance of the ligament with little discernable fibers (Fig. 14). Partial tears may be present when focal or diffuse high signal or laxity is seen to the otherwise intact tendon. ACL cysts, or idiopathic distention of the ligament with mucinous fluid, may also pose diagnostic confusion (Fig. 15). Normal striations may be obscured and a swollen or drumstick type appearance of the ACL may be seen on sagittal images. Coronal or axial images may show more of a rounded contour of high signal surrounded by intact ligament. Clinically, these patients should not have instability but may complain of knee fullness. MR imaging shows indications in the patient post-ACL reconstruction if instability or concern for repeat tear is present. A repaired ligament is taut, and a potential mimic of the pathologic condition is the possible

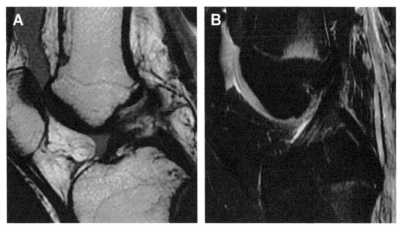

Fig. 14. Complete ACL tear. Sagittal PD-weighted image shows complete ACL tear (*arrow*), with an explosive appearance of disrupted fibers and associated joint effusion. For comparison, a sagittal PD-weighted image with fat suppression in a different patient (*B*) with a normal intact ACL was observed. The appearance of tear is contrasted with ACL degeneration in **Fig. 15**.

increased T2W signal on sagittal images, particularly in the first 2 years after reconstruction. The angle of the reconstruction tunnel should be parallel to the roof of the intercondylar notch. An imprecise tunnel angle may lead to either graft impingement if too steep or joint laxity if too shallow.

The PCL is normally low in signal in the intercondylar notch with a hooked or candy cane appearance. Tears are uncommon and not necessarily

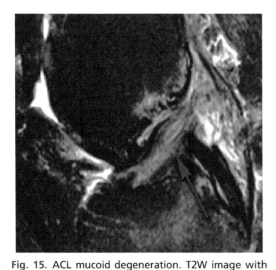

Fig. 15. ACL mucoid degeneration. T2W image with fat suppression shows intact fibers of the ACL (confirmed on serial images) with diffuse, mildly increased signal and ligamentous thickening consistent with so-called mucoid degeneration (*arrow*). Differentiation from tear may be difficult occasionally.

surgically repaired (**Fig. 16**). Tears may pose a confusing imaging appearance in that the actual disruption of fibers is not evident but rather has a stretched or drooping configuration. This somewhat nonintuitive appearance of a tear may lead to its overlook. An outright avulsion of the ligament is more obvious but rarely encountered. There may be gray signal on T1W or PD sequences but usually not high T2W signal. An analysis of PCL width on sagittal images shows torn ligaments to most often be 7 mm or thicker and normal tendons to be typically 6 mm or thinner. Abnormal signal on PD-weighted images in conjunction with a thickened ligament is suggestive of tear.[10]

The MCL courses from the medial femoral condyle to medial tibia and is interlaced with the joint capsule with direct attachments to the medial meniscus. Injuries to the MCL are common with valgus stress in sports. Edema in the region of the MCL may also be related to atraumatic causes such as osteoarthritis or may be secondary to medial meniscus tears.[13] Three grades of injury with corresponding MR imaging appearances have been described. Grade 1 or sprain is a high signal medial to the MCL in the soft tissues. Grade 2 shows high signal medially to the MCL along with partial disruption (**Fig. 17**). Grade 3 shows complete ligamentous disruption. MCL tears are generally not repaired unless in the course of repairs to other ligaments for postrepair stabilization. Fluid between the MCL and medial meniscus is diagnostic of meniscocapsular separation (**Fig. 18**), which is an important differentiation to make from an MCL sprain because the meniscocapsular separation requires immobilization to

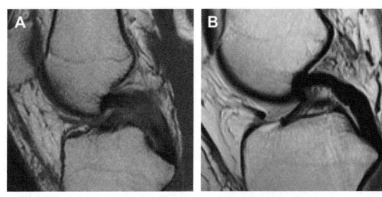

Fig. 16. Torn and normal PCL. Sagittal PD-weighted images in 2 separate patients show a thickened torn PCL (*A*) compared with an intact ligament (*B*). Thickening and intermediate signal may be the only signs of tear; findings are potentially overlooked when signs are subtler than those in this example.

allow proper healing of the peripheral vascularized meniscus.

The lateral collateral ligament (LCL) complex is made up of 3 major structures seen well at MR imaging, from anterior to posterior: iliotibial band, fibulocollateral ligament, and biceps femoris tendon. LCL tears often accompany injury to other structures in the so-called posterolateral corner. The arcuate ligament and popliteofibular ligament are important components of this structure, which may be evaluated on MR imaging. The arcuate ligament is Y shaped, which connects from the fibular styloid process to the lateral femoral condyle, with the additional limb attaching to the lateral joint capsule. Tear of the arcuate ligament is presumed when there is capsular disruption at the lateral joint line. The popliteofibular ligament is a strong lateral stabilizer of the knee. It is seen just beneath the lateral geniculate vessels on coronal images. Sagittally, the ligament is seen just superficial to the popliteus tendon. A posterolateral corner injury can be defined as a tear to a component of the LCL complex with tears of the popliteus tendon, arcuate ligament, popliteofibular ligament, and either the ACL or PCL. This injury results in pain and instability with knee hyperextension and is an indication for surgery. Knowledge of this detailed anatomy is key for making this important diagnosis.[14] Iliotibial band friction syndrome or iliotibial band syndrome may be the source of anterolateral knee pain in runners or other endurance athletes.[15] This condition may

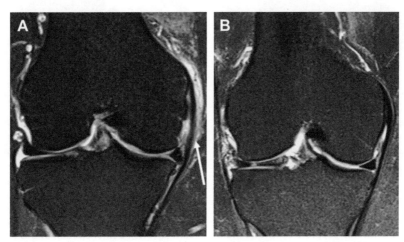

Fig. 17. MCL, partial tear and normal. Coronal PD images with fat suppression in different patients. (*A*) A grade 2 MCL sprain with some disrupted fibers and surrounding fluid signal (*B*) is compared with an intact normal MCL. The presence of high signal around the MCL does not always indicate ligamentous injury, with other differential considerations as discussed earlier.

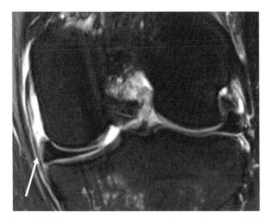

Fig. 18. Meniscocapsular separation. Coronal T2W image with fat suppression shows fluid signal tracking between the MCL and peripheral body of the medial meniscus (*arrow*). This finding was present on sequential images confirming a meniscocapsular separation. This injury is more serious than an MCL sprain.

clinically mimic a lateral meniscus tear and MR imaging can make this differentiation. Typical findings are fluid on both sides of the iliotibial band. If fluid is only seen deep to the band, it may be impossible to differentiate from joint fluid. Axial images often display this pathologic condition well (**Fig. 19**).

EXTENSOR MECHANISM/PATELLA

Lateral dislocation of the patella is an injury that because of its spontaneous reduction may be difficult for a patient to properly convey to a clinician and can be clinically difficult to separate from other internal derangements by the time of evaluation. The injury pattern is manifested on MR imaging by a typical contusion pattern along the anterior lateral femoral condyle with or without a kissing contusion of the medial patella. Dislocation disrupts the medial retinaculum (**Fig. 20**). When encountering this injury on MR imaging, integrity of the patellar cartilage must be carefully scrutinized. Cartilage defects may need surgical management. The cartilage lesion most often involves the patella but can also affect the anterior aspect of the lateral femoral condyle. A shallow trochlear groove best identified on axial images can predispose to patellar dislocation.[16]

MR imaging may be used to evaluate for patella alta or baja. A ratio of patellar length to patellar tendon length on sagittal MR images of greater than 1.5 can define patellar alta. A ratio less than 0.74 can define patellar baja.[17] Patellar baja can be associated with quadriceps tendon tears and Osgood-Schlatter disease. Patellar alta can be associated with patellofemoral dysfunction and osteoarthritis as well as predispose to patellar

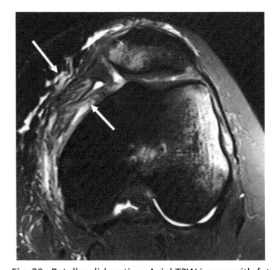

Fig. 20. Patellar dislocation. Axial T2W image with fat suppression shows typical contusion pattern of a medial patellar dislocation and relocation with edema in the lateral femoral condyle and medial aspect of patella. The medial retinaculum is also torn (*arrows*). Demonstration of this tear may be difficult at imaging and may be inferred when accompanied by the other findings of this injury. In this patient, a shallow trochlea is seen, predisposing to dislocation.

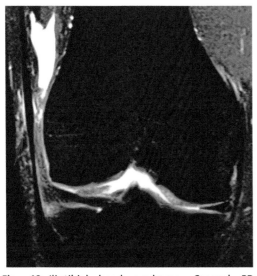

Fig. 19. Iliotibial band syndrome. Coronal PD-weighted image with fat suppression shows fluid signal surrounding the iliotibial band (*arrow*), suggestive of the iliotibial band syndrome. If fluid is only seen medially to the band, it simply may be joint fluid and does not indicate this syndrome.

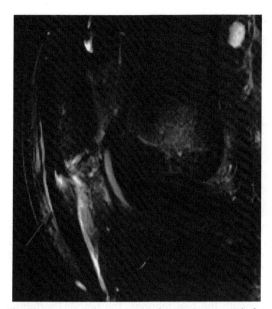

Fig. 21. Jumper's knee. Sagittal T2W image with fat suppression shows high signal, thickening, and partial tear in the patellar tendon (*arrow*), which when accompanied by anterior knee pain is consistent with jumper's knee. The clinical findings are critical for diagnosis as in other overuse syndromes because the imaging may reflect chronic changes.

dislocation. MR imaging may also identify symptomatic bipartite patellae. Bone marrow edema adjacent to the synchondrosis may be associated with correlative pain syndromes. Bipartite patellae are much more often incidental findings.

Pain inferior to the patella in athletes has been referred to as jumper's knee. MR imaging demonstrates thickening of the proximal patellar tendon with high T2W signal adjacent to the tendon (**Fig. 21**). Surgery may be required in severe cases. However, the findings can persist when patients are asymptomatic.[18]

Another source of anterior knee pain is fat pad impingement. High T2 signal in the Hoffa fat pad inferior and lateral to the patella or in the suprapatellar fat pad could indicate painful impingement of the fat pad on the femoral condyle from the patellar or quadriceps tendons. Patellar tracking abnormalities may be implicated with inferolateral fat pad signal abnormalities.

PLICAE

There are 3 major plicae in the knee, normal structures that are remnants of knee embryologic development. The plicae embryologically divided the knee into compartments. One or more of these structures may be seen on MR examinations. The medial patellar plica can be seen on axial MR images extending from the medial joint capsule toward the medial facet of the patella. Other plicae are the suprapatellar and infrapatellar plicae. These plicae may also be a source of pain syndromes. The medial patella plica may appear thickened when it is trapped between the femur and patella with recurrence and can cause clinical pain, clicking, or locking and could clinically mimic a meniscal tear. The infrapatellar plica may become thickened and a source of anterior knee

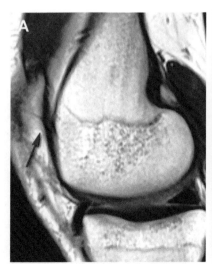
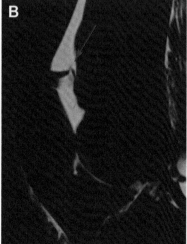

Fig. 22. Thickened plicae. (*A*) Sagittal PD-weighted image shows a thickened medial patellar plica (*arrow*). (*B*) Sagittal T2W image with fat suppression shows a thickened suprapatellar plica, creating a loculated effusion (*arrow*). Thickened, inflamed plicae may be associated with pain. In contrast, thin plicae are frequently seen at imaging and do not denote any pathologic condition.

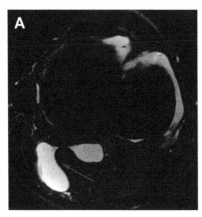
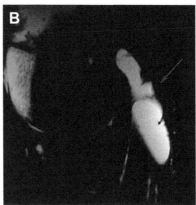

Fig. 23. Popliteus (Baker's) cyst. Axial (*A*) and sagittal (*B*) T2W images with fat suppression show a large popliteus or Baker's cyst, the most commonly encountered fluid-filled bursa about the knee (*arrows*). These bursae are most commonly present between the medial head of the gastrocnemius and semimembranosus tendons. A ruptured cyst may clinically mimic the more serious diagnosis of deep venous thrombosis.

pain in athletes (**Fig. 22**). In addition, increased T2 signal may be seen in the Hoffa fat pad along the plica's course. The definition of plica thickening is uncertain but becomes obvious in practice with experience. Inflamed thickened plicae can be readily removed with arthroscopy. Occasionally, a plica may cause mechanical friction across the articular surface leading to wear of adjacent cartilage.

BURSAE

Recognition of abnormal bursae about the knee can frequently diagnose sources of patient pain, which may mimic internal derangements that could prompt unnecessary surgery. The popliteal bursa is the most common knee bursa to show fluid signal, which is also referred to as a popliteus or Baker cyst. Baker cysts extend posteromedially from the knee between the semimembranosus and medial head of the gastrocnemius muscles (**Fig. 23**). More than 5 to 10 mL of fluid is considered potentially symptomatic and should be discussed in imaging reports. Large Baker cysts can cause compartment syndrome or lead to rupture, which may invoke inflammation in the surrounding musculature. This inflammation could mimic the more serious deep venous thrombosis.

A common cause of anterior knee pain is prepatellar bursitis, or so-called housemaid's knee. This condition usually can be a clinical diagnosis and rarely would be a sole MR imaging finding (**Fig. 24**) but can be seen in conjunction with other abnormalities. The bursa is evident if fluid is filled just superficial to the patella.

The pes anserinus bursa lies just below the knee joint line anteromedial to the tibia. The bursa lies

beneath the pes tendons, the gracilis, sartorius, and semitendinosus. If inflamed, the bursa bulges proximally toward the joint (**Fig. 25**). This bursa when inflamed may cause pain and possible clicking, mimicking a meniscal tear.

The semimembranosus-tibial collateral ligament bursa is commonly inflamed and identified on MR imaging (**Fig. 26**). This bursa is horseshoe shaped and drapes over the semimembranosus tendon along the medial joint line. It can appear to mimic a meniscal cyst extending inferiorly, but careful attention shows a lack of connection to the nearby meniscus.

An uncommonly seen bursa is the tibial collateral ligament, which is just deep to the MCL and

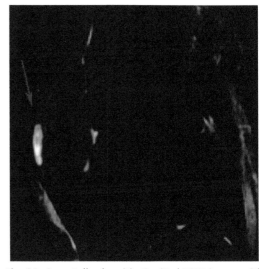

Fig. 24. Prepatellar bursitis. Sagittal T2W image with fat suppression shows high signal in the prepatellar bursa (*arrow*) compatible with bursitis.

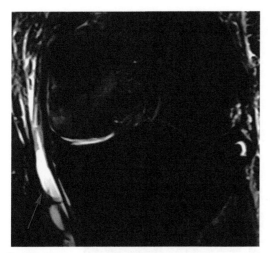

Fig. 25. Pes anserine bursitis. Coronal T2W image with fat suppression shows fluid signal in the pes anserine bursa (*arrow*) consistent with bursitis. Clinically, the symptoms may mimic a meniscal tear.

extends craniocaudally. Fluid in this bursa could be confused with a meniscocapsular separation on imaging; however, the bursa is seen to be contained and rounded, unlike the appearance of fluid related to meniscocapsular separation, which collects in the interface between the meniscus and deep surface of the MCL and capsule.

BONES

Contusions of bone (microfractures) are high in T2 signal, subarticular, and amorphous. These contusions can be a result of injury to other structures (ACL injury, patellar dislocation) but can also occur as a result of cartilage abnormalities. These microfractures can heal with appropriate rest. They may

however lead to areas of bone necrosis if large enough and not protected. Contusions that are more geographic in appearance are believed to be more at risk for such progression.

There are several described typical bone contusion patterns associated with ACL tears (discussed earlier). The most specific is the contusion of the posterolateral tibial plateau, with or without a kissing contusion of the anterior lateral femoral condyle above the anterior horn of the lateral meniscus. In severe ACL injuries, the posteromedial tibial plateau and possibly the medial femoral condyle may demonstrate contusions. It is important to recognize this contusion because the vascular peripheral meniscus may be injured or separated from the capsule.

Red marrow conversion is common about the knee and could be confused with a pathologic entity if understanding of this variant is not understood (**Fig. 27**). It is more common in women than in men and seen in higher incidence in obese smokers.[19] Red marrow is noted in the metaphysis of the femur or tibia. On T1W imaging, the signal intensity is higher in the red marrow than in the adjacent muscle.

MUSCLES/SOFT TISSUES

Tennis leg is a term coined for tears of the plantaris tendon. It may clinically resemble a tear of the medial head of the gastrocnemius with acute calf pain and skin discoloration. The plantaris muscle has its origin on the lateral femoral condyle and runs inferiorly just distal to the lateral head of the gastrocnemius and superficially to the soleus and courses deep and medial to the medial gastrocnemius running distally to the calcaneus, medial to the Achilles tendon. MR imaging can show a focal tubular fluid collection

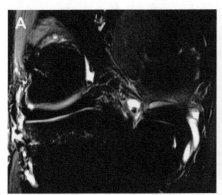
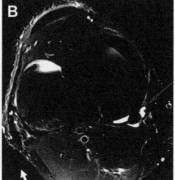

Fig. 26. Semimembranosus/tibial collateral ligament bursitis. Coronal (*A*) and axial (*B*) T2W images with fat suppression show an enlarged fluid-filled bursa along with thickening of the semimembranosus tendon (*arrows*). Occasionally, fluid in this bursa can mimic a meniscal cyst.

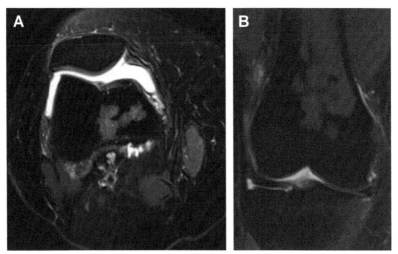

Fig. 27. Red marrow conversion in femur in an obese woman. Axial (*A*) and coronal (*B*) T2W images with fat suppression show intermediate signal where there has been red marrow conversion. This, sometimes geographic, signal can be confused with infiltrative diseases or lesions, and knowledge of appearance of red marrow in this location is important.

between the medial gastrocnemius and soleus muscles (**Fig. 28**).

Variation in the gastrocnemius muscle anatomy may cause the popliteal artery impingement syndrome and leg claudication or symptoms referable to the knee. Evaluation of the muscle belly anatomy and vascular anatomy on axial imaging is important in making the diagnosis, particularly in the proper clinical setting of vascular compromise. Diagnosis requires MR or conventional angiography, and further detail is beyond the scope of this article.[20]

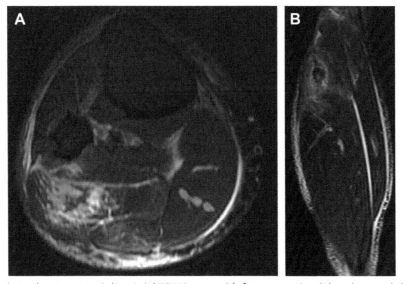

Fig. 28. Plantaris tendon tear, tennis leg. Axial T2W image with fat suppression (*A*) and coronal short tau inversion recovery image (*B*) show abnormal signal in the expected location of the plantaris tendon. A hematoma in the lateral gastrocnemius muscle is also present. These findings are characteristic of a plantaris tendon tear. Clinically, this hematoma may mimic tear in the medial head of the gastrocnemius.

SUMMARY

This article reviews useful diagnostic criteria and imaging pitfalls more commonly encountered in the knee. Knowledge of the anatomy and pathologic conditions presented can lead to more accurate and useful interpretation that can assist clinicians in patient care.

REFERENCES

1. Fox MG. MR imaging of the meniscus: review, current trends, and clinical implications. Magn Reson Imaging Clin N Am 2007;15(1):103–23.

2. De Smet AA, Norris MA, Yandow DR, et al. MR diagnosis of meniscal tears of the knee: importance of high signal in the meniscus that extends to the surface. AJR Am J Roentgenol 1993; 161(1):101–7.

3. De Smet AA, Tuite MJ. Use of the "two-slice-touch" rule for the MRI diagnosis of meniscal tears. AJR Am J Roentgenol 2006;187:911–4.

4. Helms CA, Laorr A, Cannon WD. The absent bow tie sign in bucket handle tears of the menisci of the knee. AJR Am J Roentgenol 1998;170:57–61.

5. Watt AJ, Halliday T, Raby N, et al. The value of the absent bow tie sign in MRI of bucket-handle tears. Clin Radiol 2000;55:622–6.

6. Harper KW, Helms CA, Lambert S, et al. Radial meniscal tears: significance, incidence and MR appearance. AJR Am J Roentgenol 2005;185: 1429–34.

7. Lecas L, Helms C, Kosarek F, et al. Inferiorly displaced flap tears of the medial meniscus: MR appearance and clinical significance. AJR Am J Roentgenol 2000;174:161–4.

8. De Smet A, Graf B. Meniscal tears missed on MR imaging: relationship to meniscal tear patterns and anterior cruciate ligament tears. AJR Am J Roentgenol 1994;162:905–11.

9. Singh K, Helms CA, Jacobs MT, et al. MRI appearance of Wrisberg variant of discoid lateral meniscus. AJR Am J Roentgenol 2006;187:384–7.

10. Helms C, Major N, Anderson, et al. Musculoskeletal MRI. 2nd edition. Philadelphia: Saunders; 2009.

11. Helms CA. The meniscus: recent advances in MR imaging of the knee. AJR Am J Roentgenol 2002; 179:1115–22.

12. Oei E, Nikken J, Verstignen, et al. MR imaging of the menisci and cruciate ligaments: a systematic review. Radiology 2003;226(3):837–48.

13. Wen D, Propeck T, Kane S, et al. MRI description of knee medial collateral ligament abnormalities in the absence of trauma: edema related to osteoarthritis and medial meniscal tears. Magn Reson Imaging 2007;25:209–14.

14. Vinson E, Major N, Helms C. The posterolateral corner of the knee. AJR Am J Roentgenol 2008; 190:449–58.

15. Murphy B, Hechtma K, Urie J, et al. Iliotibial band friction syndrome: MR imaging findings. Radiology 1992;185:569–71.

16. Elias D, White L, Fithian D. Acute lateral patellar dislocation at MR imaging: injury patterns of medial patellar soft tissue restraints and osteochondral injuries of the inferomedial patella. Radiology 2002; 225(3):736–43.

17. Shabshin N, Schweitzer, Morrison WB, et al. MRI criteria for patella alta and baja. Skeletal Radiol 2004;33(8):445–50.

18. Shalaby M, Almekinders L. Patellar tendinitis: the significance of magnetic resonance imaging findings. Am J Sports Med 1999;27(3):345–9.

19. Wilson A, Hodge J, Pilgrim T. Prevalence of red marrow around the knee joint in adults as demonstrated on magnetic resonance imaging. Acad Radiol 1996;3(7):550–5.

20. Radonic V, Kopic S, Giunio L, et al. Popliteal artery entrapment syndrome: diagnosis and management, with report of three cases. Tex Heart Inst J 2000; 27(1):3–13.

Normal Variants and Pitfalls in MR Imaging of the Ankle and Foot

Soterios Gyftopoulos, MD[a], Jenny T. Bencardino, MD[b],*

KEYWORDS

• MR Imaging • Ankle • Foot • Variants • Pitfalls

MR OF THE MUSCULOSKELETAL STRUCTURE

Great advances have been made in musculoskeletal radiology since the dawn of cross-sectional imaging more than three decades ago. Innovation in imaging technology has provided an unprecedented window into intra-articular pathology. MR imaging, in particular, has revolutionized the ability to study the anatomic details of all the components of the musculoskeletal system, including tendons, ligaments, muscles, and bones as well as the pathologic processes that affect them. Crucial to the accurate analysis of these structures is a solid knowledge of the anatomic variants that can be misinterpreted for pathology on MR imaging. This article focuses on the variants and imaging pitfalls in the ankle and foot.

TECHNICAL FACTORS

As a general rule, the tendons and ligaments of the ankle and foot, due to their highly organized architecture and collagen composition, demonstrate homogeneously hypointense signal on all pulse sequences. Loss of the expected low intrasubstance signal in a tendon or ligament is considered the hallmark in the diagnosis of pathologic conditions. The magic angle phenomenon is a technical phenomenon that can mimic pathology. The magic angle effect occurs when the orientation of the collagen fibers approximates the magic angle of 55° with the main magnetic vector (Z axis). This phenomenon is particularly prominent when a low echo time (TE) of 10 to 20 milliseconds is used, as in T1-weighted, proton density, and gradient-echo sequences. T2-weighted or short tau inversion recovery (STIR) images with high TE values (>35 milliseconds) eliminate the magic angle effect. When imaging the ankle, this phenomenon can be reduced by scanning patients in the prone position or positioning the foot at 20° of plantar flexion while scanning patients in a supine position. The magic angle more frequently affects the posterior tibial tendon just proximal to its navicular insertion, the peroneal tendons in subfibular position, and the anterior tendons at the level of the ankle joint (**Figs. 1 and 2**).

Incomplete fat suppression can falsely produce hyperintense signal in the soft tissues and bone marrow, most commonly in the lateral aspect of the ankle in the region of the lateral malleolus, although the medial malleolus can also be affected (**Fig. 3**). This is thought to be due to factors, such as coil proximity artifact and the presence of inhomogeneities in the static magnetic field. Inhomogeneous fat saturation can be combated through the use of inversion recovery imaging, which is insensitive to field inhomogenities, and by the use of multichannel phase array coils.

TENDONS
Anterior Compartment

The anterior compartment tendons (anterior tibial, extensor hallucis longus, extensor digitorum longus, and peroneus tertius) are rarely injured. The anterior tibial tendon is the most commonly injured

[a] Department of Radiology, NYU Hospital for Joint Diseases, New York, NY 10003, USA
[b] Department of Radiology, NYU Hospital for Joint Diseases, 310 East 17th Street Sixth Floor, New York, NY 10003, USA
* Corresponding author.
E-mail address: Jenny.bencardino@nyumc.org

Magn Reson Imaging Clin N Am 18 (2010) 691–705
doi:10.1016/j.mric.2010.07.007

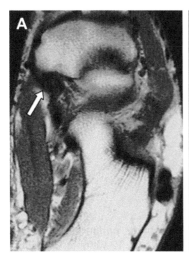
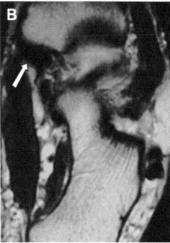

Fig. 1. Magic angle phenomenon is demonstrated on the axial T1-weighted image (A) as intrasubstance intermediate signal within the insertional fibers of the posterior tibial tendon (white arrow), which entirely disappears on the fast spin-echo T2-weighted image (B).

extensor tendon. Tear of the anterior tibial tendon is classically seen in older patients and athletes who run hills.[1] Apparent longitudinal split tearing in the insertional portion of this tendon at the medial cuneiform bone and base of the first metatarsal in asymptomatic patients is most likely related to the presence of multiple insertional slips. This is thought to represent a normal variant.[2]

Medial Compartment

The insertional portion of the posterior tibial tendon on the medial navicular tubercle typically has a heterogenous appearance. This signal heterogeneity is secondary to a combination of magic angle effect and fat interposed between the insertional slips of the tendon.[3,4] Another cause of the heterogeneity is the presence of an intratendinous accessory navicular bone (type I

accessory navicular bone [os tibiale externum]) (**Fig. 4**).[5]

A small amount of tenosynovial fluid is frequently observed within the tendon sheaths in asymptomatic individuals and should not be considered abnormal. Physiologic tenosynovial fluid is more frequently found in the flexor than in the extensor tendons.[6] The lack of tendon sheath in the distal preinsertional portion of the posterior tibial tendon renders fluid signal in this location abnormal, however. Posterior tibial peritendinitis likely related to metaplastic synovium should be considered.[6] Disproportionate fluid within the flexor tendon sheaths, compared with the amount of fluid found in the ankle joint, is usually indicative of tenosynovitis. Communication between the ankle joint and the flexor hallucis longus tendon, however, explains the presence of prominent fluid within this tendon sheath in patients with large joint effusions. Thus, even a large amount of fluid within

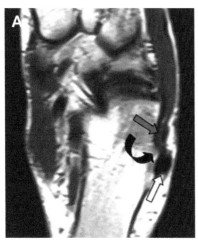
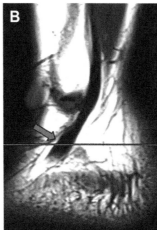

Fig. 2. Axial proton density (A) and sagittal T1-weighted (B) images demonstrate high signal within the peroneus brevis tendon (gray arrow) at the level of the peroneal tubercle (curved arrow) of the lateral calcaneal wall related to magic angle phenomenon (arrows). The peroneus longus tendon (white arrow) is not affected because it is coursing more vertically with respect to the peroneus brevis tendon at this level.

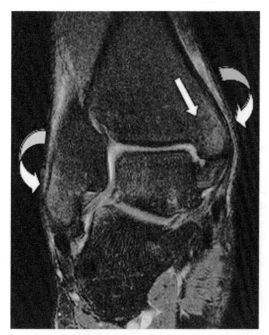

Fig. 3. Coronal, fat-suppressed, T2-weighted image of the ankle demonstrates inhomogenous fat suppression resulting in spurious increased signal in the lateral and medial malleoli and overlying soft tissues (*arrows*).

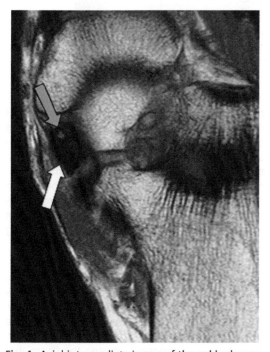

Fig. 4. Axial intermediate image of the ankle demonstrates a type I accessory navicular (*gray arrow*) embedded within the posterior tibial tendon (*white arrow*).

the tendon sheath of the flexor hallucis longus tendon may be of no clinical significance.[6]

Posterior Compartment

The tendons of the gastrocnemius and soleus muscles form the Achilles tendon. The Achilles tendon measures approximately 15 cm in length and typically has a fascicular appearance secondary to the intermixing of its fibers with fibrofatty tissue and vessels. This, in turn, produces intrasubstance linear and punctate hyperintense foci on T1-weighted and gradient-echo images.[7] Preservation of the normal morphology of the tendon helps differentiate this signal heterogeneity from a partial tear because a normal tendon maintains its normal flat/concave shape anteriorly and demonstrates intact fibers throughout its course without intervening fluid-like T2 signal. In addition, the fascicular appearance is usually less apparent on STIR and T2-weighted images.[8,9]

Low or incomplete incorporation of the gastrocnemius and soleus tendons may produce heterogeneity due to persistent fat planes between the tendon slips. Assessment of the course of the soleus tendon relative to the gastrocnemius tendon on sequential axial images avoids confusing this normal variant with disease (**Fig. 5**).[10] A pathologic process that can mimic this appearance is a xanthomatous Achilles tendon. Xanthomas are composed of lipid-filled foamy histiocytes and extracellular cholesterol deposits. They are typically seen in patients with inherited metabolic diseases, such as familial hypercholesterolemia and hyperproteinemia.[11,12] A xanthomatous Achilles tendon typically has a speckled or reticulated appearance with or without tendon enlargement.[12] This MR imaging appearance correlated with a patient's medical history helps diagnose this pathologic process.

Lateral Compartment

The peroneal tendons (peroneus brevis and peroneus longus) share a common tendon sheath down to the level of the lateral malleolar tip. From this point on, the tendons have individual tendon sheaths. The peroneal tendons can be affected by magic angle effect because they course obliquely around the lateral malleolus and onto their insertions in the foot, particularly as the peroneus longus tendon curves beneath the cuboid bone. The primary restraints to subluxation of the peroneal tendons are the superior and inferior peroneal retinacula. The superior peroneal retinaculum courses from the posterolateral aspect of the distal fibula to the lateral calcaneus and helps stabilize the tendons in the retromalleolar groove.

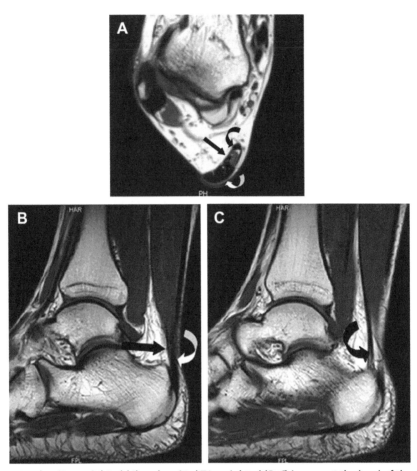

Fig. 5. Axial proton density—weighted (*A*) and sagittal T1-weighted (*B, C*) images at the level of the distal Achilles tendon (*curved white arrow*) demonstrates a low incorporating soleus (*straight arrow*) as well as a separate accessory soleus tendon (*curved black arrow*) inserting into the posteromedial calcaneus.

The inferior peroneal retinaculum attaches to the peroneal trochlea and calcaneus above and below the tendons while forming a septum that reinforces the individual tendon sheaths. The oblique course of the peroneus brevis tendon leads to apparent subluxation of the tendon where the brevis tendon is found medial to the medial margin of the fibular groove instead of at its more frequent position posterior to the fibular groove and anterior to the peroneus longus tendon. Pseudosubluxation of the peroneus brevis tendon can be further accentuated in foot supination.[13]

LIGAMENTS
Lateral Compartment

Of the three main ligaments in the low lateral compartment of the ankle, the least prone to injury is the posterior talofibular ligament. This ligament tends to have a fan-like, striated appearance on MR imaging that should not be confused with

a sprain or tear.[4,14] The posterior talofibular ligament and the posterior intermalleolar ligament course transversely posterior to the tibiotalar joint and, thus, frequently appear as punctuate hypointensities as they are imaged in cross section in the sagittal plane. This appearance can mimic posterior ankle intra-articular bodies. It is important to carefully track each of these ligaments from their origin to insertion to exclude the presence of a loose body using the orthogonal imaging planes.[4,14]

Syndesmotic Ligaments

The anterior tibiofibular ligament can also pose a diagnostic dilemma, because it may appear thickened and discontinuous. This appearance can be a normal finding and is thought to be related to fat interposed between the fibers that make up the ligament as well as due to its downward oblique orientation from the anterior tibial lip to its insertion into the fibular malleolus

(Fig. 6). As with the posterior intermalleolar and posterior talofibular ligaments (discussed previously), the anterior and posterior tibiofibular ligaments can mimic intra-articular loose bodies on the sagittal plane due to their transverse course.[4,14]

Medial Compartment

The deltoid ligament complex is made up of superficial and deep layers. One of the most readily visualized components of the complex is the posterior tibiotalar ligament, a component of the deep layer. This ligament has a striated appearance due to the presence of intervening fat between its fibers, which should not be confused with injury. This striated appearance is regularly seen in the young adult population.[4,14,15]

The spring ligament complex is made up of three separate components: the superomedial, the medial plantar oblique, and the inferior plantar longitudinal fibers. The spring ligament complex is an important structure of the anterior subtalar joint providing a fibrocartilaginous articular surface to the talar head (Fig. 7A). The superomedial component, which courses from the medial aspect of the sustentaculum tali to the superomedial aspect of the navicular, runs medial to the distal posterior tibial tendon and is separated by loose connective tissue.[16] This loose connective tissue helps differentiate between the posterior tibial tendon and superomedial spring ligament. Frequently noted between the medial plantar oblique and the inferior plantar longitudinal ligaments is a fluid-filled recess of the talocalcaneonavicular (Fig. 7B). Fluid signal within this recess may potentially be misconstrued as a spring ligament tear. Visualization of the recess is facilitated by the presence of a native effusion or by intra-articular injection of contrast solution in the talonavicular joint. Posttraumatic talonavicular effusions in the setting of acute impaction injury of the talar head and talonavicular osteoarthritis are often seen in association with a fluid distended spring recess.[17]

Accessory Ligaments

The posterior intermalleolar ligament is a ligament found in the posterior aspect of the ankle in 81.8% of specimens.[18] It was originally described as a ligamentous structure extending between the medial malleolus and the lateral malleolus (Fig. 8). Recent studies have reported a diverse group of medial origins with the lateral insertion consistently found in the medial fossa of the lateral malleolus.[18] This ligament can have different shapes depending on the site of its medial origin as well as of the number of fiber bundles and their density. The posterior intermalleolar ligament can potentially become entrapped and be a cause of posterior ankle impingement.[19]

In general, it is important to correlate the clinical history along with the imaging findings when evaluating these structures for injury. The morphology of each ligament and tendon should be carefully examined as well as its signal in conjunction with the status of the surrounding soft tissue and osseous structures to confidently differentiate a tear or sprain from a normal variant.

MUSCLES

Muscle variants are frequently seen in the ankle.[4,14,20,21] These muscles are usually asymptomatic and often incidentally found on MR imaging obtained for unrelated reasons. When they do come to attention, they can either present as a mass on physical examination or cause pain related to their effect on the surrounding structures.[20,21] For instance, the peroneal tunnel can house an accessory muscle, the peroneus quartus, which is located adjacent to the peroneus brevis and peroneus longus tendons. This muscle can cause peroneal tunnel overcrowding, leading to

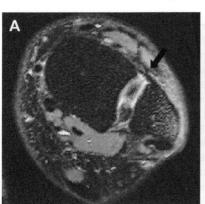
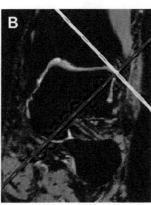

Fig. 6. Axial, oblique, fat-suppressed, proton density, 3-D reconstructed image (A) demonstrates the anterior tibiofibular ligament in its entirety (arrow). (B) Coronal, oblique, proton density, source 3-D image.

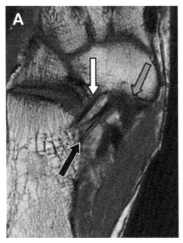 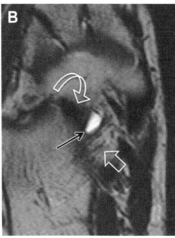

Fig. 7. (*A*) Axial intermediate-weighted image of the ankle demonstrates the medioplantar oblique (*black arrow*) and infero-plantar longitudinal (*white arrow*) components of the spring liga-ment complex normally found at the level of the posterior tibial tendon attachment on the medial navicular tubercle (*gray arrow*). (*B*) Axial fast spin echo T2-weighted image demonstrates a fluid filled spring ligament recess (*black arrow*) interposed between the medioplantar oblique (*open arrow*) and inferoplantar longitu-dinal (*curve arrow*) components.

mass effect and compression on the peroneus brevis and peroneus longus tendons and eventual tearing.[22] The peroneus quartus inserts indepen-dently into the retrotrochlear eminence of the lateral calcaneus, which helps differentiate it from a low-lying peroneus brevis muscle belly (**Fig. 9**). The latter, unlike the peroneus quartus, does not predispose to tearing. The flexor acces-sorius digitorum longus (FADL) is the most common accessory muscle found within the tarsal tunnel. Due to its location inside the tarsal tunnel, the FADL can cause mass effect on the adjacent tibial nerve or its plantar branches, particularly during exercise-related engorgement leading to neuropathy and denervation (**Fig. 10**).[23] Other common normal muscle variants include the accessory soleus,[24,25] low incorporation of the

soleus, and peroneo calcaneus internus muscles. An accessory soleus can be distinguished from low incorporation of the soleus by following the course of the tendon in question. The tendon of the accessory soleus inserts separately onto the calcaneus anteromedial to the attachment of the Achilles.[26]

BONES

There are various normal anatomic variants and pitfalls related to the osseous structures of the ankle and foot. Similar to the evaluation of the liga-ments and tendons, it is important to not only be familiar with these variants but also use the infor-mation in the surrounding structures to make an accurate diagnosis.

Os Variants

Ossicles or secondary ossifications centers can be found in various locations of the foot and ankle. They are usually asymptomatic, but it is important to not confuse them with a fracture fragment or tumor of osseous origin. This can be avoided by knowing their typical location, configuration, and size.

In the medial ankle compartment, the most frequently found accessory ossicle is the os navi-culare. Three types have been described, each with its own characteristic imaging appearance and clinical significance.[27] A type I accessory navicular ossicle or os tibiale externum is found embedded in the distal portion of the posterior tibial tendon. It has a round or oval shape, can measure between 2 to 6 mm in diameter, and is usually located up to 5 mm proximal to the medial navicular tubercle (see **Fig. 4**). A type I accessory navicular is typically of no clinical significance. The ossicle typically follows the MR imaging

Fig. 8. Coronal intermediate-weighted image demon-strating the posterior intermalleolar ligament (*curved white arrow*) extending from the posterior margin of the medial malleolus (*star*) to the lateral malleolar fovea (*black arrow*) interposed between the inferior band of the posterior tibiofibular ligament (*gray arrow*) and the posterior talofibular ligament (*white arrow*).

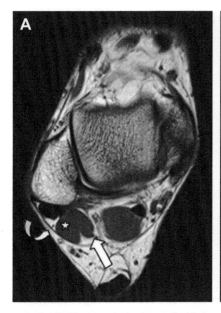

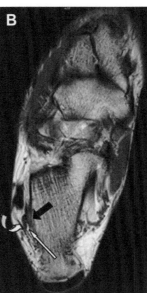

Fig. 9. Axial intermediate-weighted images (*A, B*) demonstrate a peroneus quartus muscle (*white arrow*) descending within the peroneal tunnel along the medial aspect of the peroneus brevis muscle (*asterisk*). Note the conjoint insertion of the peroneus quartus onto the retrotrochlear eminence (*black arrow*) with the inferior peroneal retinaculum (*curved white arrow*).

characteristics of bone marrow with a thin cortical hypointense margin. A type II accessory navicular ossicle has a triangular shape, and is attached to the medial navicular via a cartilaginous and/or fibrous syndesmosis. It can serve as the main site of attachment for the posterior tibial tendon, which in turn, may cause stress at the synchondrosis. This can present, clinically, as medial-sided midfoot pain. MR imaging can demonstrate T2 hyperintense signal within the synchondrosis, accessory navicular, medial navicular tuberosity, and surrounding soft tissues, representing edema, in what is known as symptomatic accessory navicular syndrome.[4,28] A type III accessory ossicle has a complete osseous fusion and incorporation to

the navicular bone, creating a horn-like or cornuate navicular. This type of ossicle serves as an attachment site for the posterior tibial tendon reducing the distance between the lateral malleolus fulcrum and the medial navicular insertion. This is thought to increase biomechanical stress in the tendon fibers, increasing the risk of tendinosis and tear (**Fig. 11**).[29]

The lateral compartment contains the os peroneum, an accessory ossicle embedded within the tendon of the peroneus longus tendon. This ossicle is regularly seen in primates related to the peroneus longus tendon role in hallux adduction.[30] In humans, the os peroneum is found in 20% of the population and serves no functional purpose.[31]

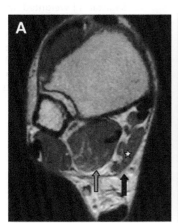

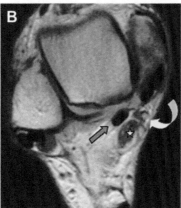

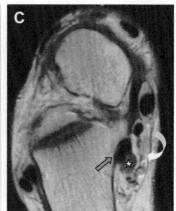

Fig. 10. Axial proton density–weighted images (*A–C*) of the ankle demonstrate an accessory flexor digitorum longus (*asterisk*) emanating proximally from the flexor retinaculum (*black arrow*) and extending alongside to the flexor hallucis longus muscle and tendon (*gray arrow*) and posterior neurovascular bundle (*curved arrow*).

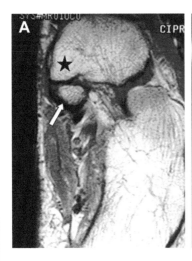
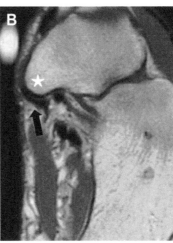

Fig. 11. Axial intermediate images demonstrate a type II navicular (*arrow*) articulating to the medial navicular tubercle (*star*) (*A*) and the posterior tibial tendon (*black arrow*) inserting onto a cornuate navicular (*white star*) (*B*).

This ossicle is bipartite or tripartite in 25% of cases.[32] Painful os peroneum syndrome presents clinically as tenderness along the lateral side of the foot at the level of the calcaneocuboid joint and is characterized on MR imaging by edematous changes in the ossicle and surrounding tendon fibers. It has a variety of causes, including fracture, peroneus longus tendon tear, and entrapment by an enlarged peroneal tubercle.[33]

Differentiation between a multipartite os peroneum and fractured os peroneum can be difficult. An acute fracture would demonstrate edematous changes in the ossicle and surrounding soft tissues. The fracture fragments have noncorticated, irregular margins, and the fragments should be able to fit together into the normal form and size of a regular os peroneum. The moieties of the multipartite os peroneum should have well corticated, smooth margins and the sum of the moieties would result in a much larger ossicle.

The os trigonum is found in the region of the posterior lateral talar tubercle. This ossicle usually forms a fibrocartilaginous syndesmosis with the talus and first becomes mineralized between the ages of 7 and 13. The ossification usually fuses with the talus to form the lateral tubercle of posterior talar process (Stieda process) but can remain a separate ossicle in 7% to 14% of people (**Fig. 12**).[34,35] Os trigonum syndrome is seen in patients who take part in activities that involve extreme plantar flexion, such as ballet, football, and soccer. The syndrome presents clinically with chronic posterior ankle pain, stiffness, and swelling due to the impingement of synovial and capsular tissue in between the posterior calcaneus, the os trigonum, and the posterior tibia.

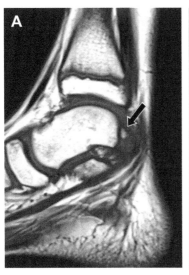
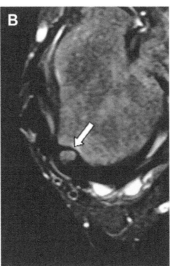

Fig. 12. Sagittal T1-weighted (*A*) and axial, fat-suppressed, T2-weighted (*B*) images demonstrate an unfused os trigonum in a skeletally immature patient (*arrows*). Note normal signal intensity within the ossification center and its synchondrosis.

MR imaging may reveal edematous changes in the posterior ankle capsule and ligaments as well as within the ossicle and posterior talus. The flexor hallucis longus tendon travels between the os trigonum and the posterior medial talar tubercle and can become inflamed, leading to chronic changes of tendinosis and/or stenosing tenosynovitis.[34] It may also be difficult to distinguish an os trigonum from a fracture of the posterior lateral talar tubercle. The irregular margins of a fracture fragment and related posttraumatic soft tissue changes can be seen on MR and CT imaging, helping distinguish between an os trigonum and a fracture of the posterior lateral talar tubercle (**Fig. 13**).[34,36]

The os intermetatarseum is an accessory ossicle found in the dorsal aspect of the midfoot between the bases of the first and second metatarsals. It can have several different shapes, including round, oval, spindle, and linear. The os intermetatarseum can form a synovial-lined joint with or become fused to an adjacent bone. Although it rarely can become symptomatic, its true importance lies in its ability to mimic a small fracture related to a Lisfranc injury. When evaluating a possible Lisfranc injury, it is important to look for other related findings, including dorsal soft tissue swelling and malalignment that help decipher between these entities.[37] The os intermetatarseum can also lead to impingement of the deep peroneal nerve as it travels dorsal to the first proximal intermetatarsal space.

The os sustentaculi is a rare accessory ossicle found at the posterior end of the sustentaculum tali along the medial aspect of the calcaneus. There is usually a fibrous or fibrocartilaginous bridge between the os sustentaculi and the calcaneus. It is best depicted in the coronal and axial planes. Familiarity with the presence of the os sustentaculi avoids the misdiagnosis of a fracture or unusual exostosis.[38]

Sesamoids

The tibial (medial) and fibular (lateral) hallucal sesamoids are found in the tendon slips of the flexor hallucis brevis and abductor hallucis muscles. Their size and shape may vary with the tibial sesamoid tending to be more elliptical whereas the fibular sesamoid tends to be more cylindrical in shape. Although both sesamoids can be partitioned, the tibial sesamoid is more frequently so. Although it has been theorized that the partitioning is due to remote trauma before ossification, this is usually a normal appearance not to be confused with fracture.[39] Bipartite hallucal ossicles have smooth and well-defined corticated margins. The sum of the proximal and distal moieties of bipartite hallucal sesamoids produces a larger-sized ossicle, which helps to distinguish a bipartite sesamoid from a fractured sesamoid. Bipartite sesamoids may be more prone to stress-related changes, including marrow edema-like pattern, fractures, and avascular necrosis.[40]

Osseous Landmarks

The retromalleolar groove is a normal shallow concavity found along the posterior aspect of the distal fibula approximately 1 cm above the tibiotalar joint that accommodates the peroneal tendons as they travel from the ankle into the foot.[41] The shape of the groove can vary from flat (11%) to convex (7%). Nonconcave shapes are thought to predispose to peroneal tendon pathology, including lateral dislocations and longitudinal tears.[42] In a recent study in asymptomatic volunteers, convex, flat, or irregular retromalleolar grooves were found in up to 72% of cases without evidence of tendon pathology.[43] Although the role

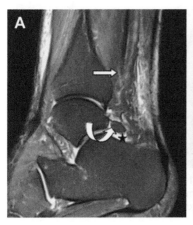
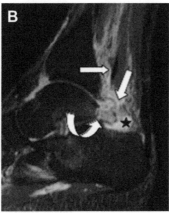

Fig. 13. (*A*) Sagittal, fat-suppressed, T2-weighted image demonstrates an os trigonum (*curved white arrow*) in an adult patient exhibiting normal internal marrow signal. Note fluid in the posterior subtalar joint recess (*asterisk*) and normal flexor hallucis longus tendon (*straight white arrow*). (*B*) Oblique, sagittal, STIR image shows a markedly edematous os trigonum (*curved arrow*) associated with posterior subtalar joint effusion (*asterisk*) as well as flexor hallucis longus strain and tenosynovitis (*straight white arrows*).

of the retromalleolar groove is in question, the authors believe it is still important to carefully evaluate the peroneal tendons and the superior peroneal retinaculum for peroneal tendon dysfunction and superior peroneal retinacular injury whenever a nonconcave fibular retromalleolar groove is encountered.

The lateral wall of the calcaneus may have an undulating configuration due to the presence of two osseous protuberances. Along the anterior aspect of the lateral calcaneal wall, the peroneal tubercle can be seen in 40% of normal individuals contributing to the peroneal tendon fibro-osseous wall along the calcaneus (**Fig. 14**). More posteriorly, a more broad-based retrotrochlear eminence is seen in 98% of the general population (**Fig. 15**). These osseous structures can grow overtime and cause problems for patients and radiologists. A hypertrophied peroneal tubercle or retrotrochlear eminence can mimic an osteochondroma or even a healing fracture. A prominent peroneal tubercle can cause mechanical friction on the adjacent peroneal longus tendon and/or peroneus brevis tendon, leading to tears and/or tenosynovitis.[44] In addition, symptomatic adventitial bursitis may develop in the vicinity of the peroneal trochlea and/or retrotrochlear eminence.[45]

Pseudocoalition

The two most common coalitions in the ankle are the subtalar and calcaneonavicular types. The coalitions can be fibrous, cartilaginous, or osseous in nature. Tarsal coalitions can be sources of chronic ankle and foot pain. The subtalar coalition is often seen at the middle subtalar joint and can be differentiated from the normal joint by its irregular opposing margins and its medial to lateral downward slope (**Fig. 16**). In addition, the sustentaculum talus tends to be deformed. True subtalar coalition should be distinguished from pseudo-coalition of the medial subtalar joint.[4] A subtalar pseudocoalition is depicted on coronal and sometimes axial images as an osseous bar between the talus and the calcaneus, which is traversed by a vague, low-signal, linear shadow migrating from a cranial to caudal location on sequential images (**Fig. 17**). This appearance reflects partial volume averaging generated by the obliquity of

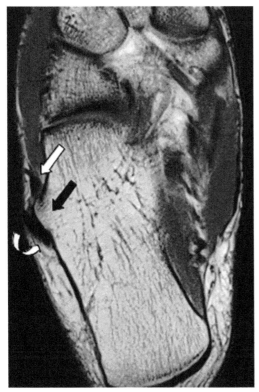

Fig. 14. Axial proton density–weighted image demonstrates an enlarged peroneal tubercle (*black arrow*) interposed between the peroneus brevis tendon (*white arrow*) and the peroneus longus tendon (*curved arrow*).

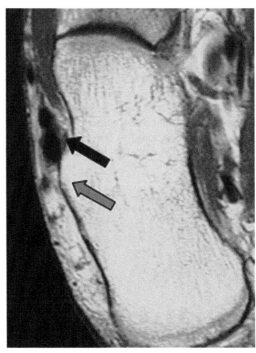

Fig. 15. Axial T1-weighted image of the ankle demonstrates a retromalleolar tubercle (*gray arrow*) along the posteromedial aspect of the peroneal tendons (*black arrow*).

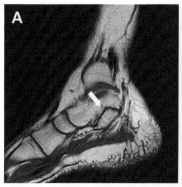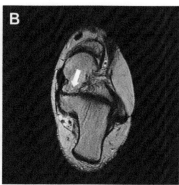

Fig. 16. Sagittal T1-weighted (A) and axial (B) fast spin-echo T2-weighted images demonstrate a fibrous subtalar coalition affecting the middle facets of the talus and calcaneus (*arrows*).

the medial subtalar joint relative to the orthogonal coronal or axial planes. This partial volume averaging is not infrequently encountered on routine axial CT images. The presence of a normal medial subtalar joint and sustentaculum talus on sagittal MR images aids in distinguishing a pseudocoalition from true coalition.

An osseous coalition between the calcaneus and the navicular bone is often simulated on sagittal T1-weighted images of the hindfoot. This pitfall can be easily avoided by noting a normal relationship between the two bones on axial and coronal images. Also, in the absence of a true coalition, gradient-echo or STIR sagittal images demonstrate bright signal between the calcaneus and navicular precluding the existence of a calcaneonavicular bar (**Fig. 18**).

The presence of a normal articulation between the navicular and cuboid has been reported in up to 45% of cadaveric ankles.[46] Therefore, the presence of articulating margins on axial images between the navicular and the cuboid should not be interpreted as coalition. This is in contradistinction to the calcaneus and navicular, which should not have articulating margins on axial images.

Pseudolesions

Pseudo-osteochondral defects are seen in the tibial plafond and the talus. The confluence of cortical trabeculae at the normal elevation of the posterior distal tibial articular surface can occasionally form a linear focus of hypointense signal in the far posterior coronal MR images of the plafond.[47] A normal groove located in the posterior aspect of the talus housing the posterior talofibular ligament can mimic an osteochondral lesion or erosion.[48] A curvilinear hypointense band produced by the insertion of the tibiotalar ligament onto the central talus can produce a pseudodefect in the subchondral

bone or a few millimeters below the articular surface.

The normal multifaceted, asymmetric shape of the metatarsal bases can produce apparent articular incongruency on MR imaging, leading to the false impression of subluxation, particularly at the tarsometatarsal joint. This pitfall may lead to the misdiagnosis of a Lisfranc injury.[49] Familiarity with the typical location of these pseudolesions as well as lack of associated findings, such as soft tissue or bone marrow edema, help radiologists avoid misinterpreting normal anatomy for pathology.

Bone Marrow

Marrow edema-like signal defined as focal areas of ill-defined hypointensity on T1 and bright patchy T2 signal on fluid-sensitive sequences is a nonspecific MR finding that can be secondary to several different causes, including hematopoietic marrow reconversion, infection, trauma, and tumor. Several factors need to be considered in some cases to differentiate between these various causes, including age, distribution, and adjacent soft tissue and bone findings. Foci of high T2 signal in a starry-night pattern can be seen in the talus and calcaneus in asymptomatic patients, usually below the age of 15. These foci are thought to be caused by perivascular foci of red marrow, physiologic stress, or increased bone turnover related to weight bearing or normal skeletal growth.[50,51]

High T2 signal round/ovoid foci can also be regularly seen in the anterior calcaneus at the angle of Gissane.[52] These foci are thought to represent nutrient channels or intraosseous ganglion cysts (**Fig. 19**).[53,54] Similar-appearing high T2 foci are seen in the dorsal aspect of the talar neck and along the plantar sinus tarsi surface, which are also thought to represent vessels. Finally, high T2 signal foci can also be seen at

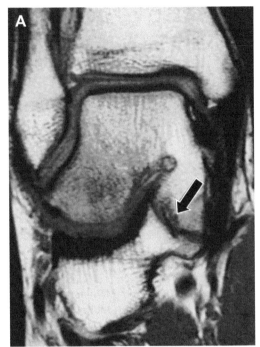

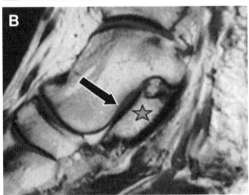

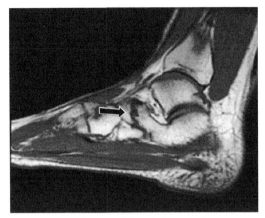

Fig. 18. Sagittal T1-weighted image demonstrates a fibrous calcaneonavicular coalition (*arrow*).

bone marrow edema should be expected by 18 weeks after immobilization.[55]

Transient Physiologic MR Imaging Findings

Bursae are anatomic cushions or sacs that facilitate motion between apposing tissues.[56] They are classified into three main types: congenital, anatomic, and adventitial. Congenital bursae develop in utero and are synovial lined. Anatomic bursae develop in children at sites of normal friction, whereas

Fig. 17. Coronal T1-weighted image (*A*) of the ankle demonstrates a low signal area traversing an osseous bar in the middle subtalar joint that gives the appearance of a coalition (*black arrow*). Note the normal middle talar (*black arrow*) and calcaneal (*star*) facets of the subtalar joint on the sagittal T1-weighted image (*B*) consistent with a pseudocoalition.

several different ligament and tendon attachments, most commonly in the posterior talus and fibular notch at the attachments of the posterior talofibular ligament (**Fig. 20**).

Bone marrow edema pattern has also been described within the first 12 weeks after immobilization treatment after an injury. This pattern was not found to correlate with new pain or the clinical syndrome of reflex sympathetic dystrophy. Resolution or stabilization of this

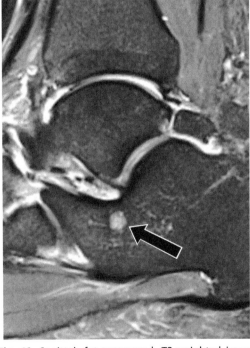

Fig. 19. Sagittal, fat-suppressed, T2-weighted image demonstrates a pseudocyst in the calcaneus just inferior to the critical angle of Gissane (*arrow*).

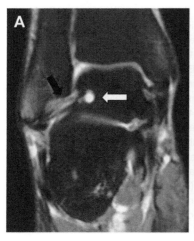

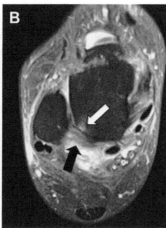

Fig. 20. (A) Coronal, fat-suppressed, T2-weighted image of the ankle demonstrate a traction cyst (*white arrow*) at the talar attachment of the posterior talofibular ligament (*black arrow*). (B) Axial, fat-suppressed, T2-weighted image demonstrates reactive marrow edema (*white arrow*) at the site of insertion of a partly torn posterior tibiofibular ligament (*black arrow*) in the setting of posterior ankle impingement.

adventitial bursae develop in adults secondary to chronic friction between soft tissues and adjacent osseous structures. Anatomic and adventitial bursae are not synovial lined. Adventitial bursae can be found throughout the foot and ankle and are usually formed adjacent to osseous protuberances.[57–61] Common locations include adjacent to the medial and lateral malleoli (**Fig. 21**), plantar surfaces of the metatarsal heads, and medial surface of the first metatarsal head. The superficial Achilles bursa is an example of an adventitial bursa that does not develop next to an osseous protuberance. Instead, it tends to develop as a result of chronic inflammation of the Achilles tendon in disorders, such as Haglund syndrome.[62] An example of a congenital bursa is the retrocalcaneal bursa, which is located between the Achilles tendon and posterosuperior aspect of the calcaneus. A small amount of physiologic fluid can be seen in this bursa normally after some activity.[63] It also can become inflamed secondary to inflammatory arthropathies, such as rheumatoid arthritis, because of its synovial lining as well as from chronic friction with the adjacent calcaneus and Achilles tendon.[60]

Transient physiologic MR imaging findings can be seen in the ankle and foot after physical activity that can mimic pathologic conditions. Fluid can be seen in the ankle joint, retrocalcaneal bursa, and the tendon sheaths, most commonly in the flexor hallucis longus. Bone marrow edema can also be occasionally present, especially after strenuous activity.[64] Physiologic fluid can be present in the first three intermetatarsal bursae in asymptomatic patients. Morton neuromas have also been found in 30% of asymptomatic subjects. It has been speculated that these neuromas

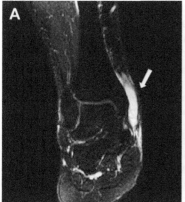

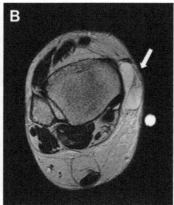

Fig. 21. Coronal, fat-suppressed, T2-weighted (A) and axial, fast spin-echo, T2-weighted (B) images demonstrate medial malleolar bursitis (*arrows*).

may only become relevant when they reach a transverse diameter of 5 mm or more. Correlation with patient clinical history and physical examination is recommended.[65,66]

REFERENCES

1. Ouzounian TJ, Anderson R. Anterior tibial tendon rupture. Foot Ankle Int 1995;16:406–10.

2. Mengiardi B, Pfirrmann CW, Vienne P, et al. Anterior tibial tendon abnormalities: MR imaging findings. Radiology 2005;235:977–84.

3. Erickson SJ, Cox IH, Hyde JS, et al. Effect of tendon orientation on MR imaging signal intensity: a manifestation of the "magic angle" phenomenon. Radiology 1991;181:389–92.

4. Rosenberg ZS, Bencardino J, Mellado JM. Normal variants and pitfalls in magnetic resonance imaging of the foot and ankle. Top Magn Reson Imaging 1998;9:262–72.

5. Delfaut EM, Demondion X, Bieganski A, et al. The fibrocartilaginous sesamoid: a cause of size and signal variation in the normal distal posterior tibial tendon. Eur Radiol 2003;13:2642–9.

6. Schweitzer ME, Van Leersum M, Ehrlich SS, et al. Fluid in normal and abnormal ankle joints: amount and distribution as seen on MR Images. Am J Roentgenol 1994;162:111–4.

7. Mantel D, Falutre B, Bastian D, et al. [Structural MRI study of the Achilles tendon: correlation with microanatomy and histology]. J Radiol 1996;77:261–5 [in French].

8. Schweitzer ME, Karasick D. MR imaging of disorders of the posterior tibial tendon. Am J Roentgenol 2000;175:627–35.

9. Soila K, Karjalainen PT, Aronen HJ, et al. High resolution MR imaging of the asymptomatic Achilles tendon: new observations. Am J Roentgenol 1999; 173:323–8.

10. Mellado JM, Rosenberg ZS, Beltran J, et al. Low incorporation of the soleus tendon: MR interpretation pitfall. Skeletal Radiol 1998;27:222–4.

11. Schweitzer ME, Karasick D. MR imaging of disorders of the Achilles tendon. Am J Roentgenol 2000;175:613–25.

12. Bude RO, Adler RS, Bassett DR. Diagnosis of Achilles Tendon Xanthoma in patients with heterozygous familial hypercholesterolemia: MR vs Sonography. Am J Roentgenol 1994;162:913–7.

13. Wang XT, Rosenberg ZS, Mechlin MB, et al. Normal variants and diseases of the peroneal tendons and superior peroneal retinaculum: MR imaging features. Radiographics 2005;25:587–602.

14. Noto AM, Cheung Y, Rosenberg ZS, et al. MR imaging of the ankle: normal variants. Radiology 1989;170:121–4.

15. Mengiardi B, Pfirrman CW, Vienne P. Medial collateral ligament complex of the ankle: MR appearance in asymptomatic subjects. Radiology 2007;242:817–24.

16. Mengiardi B, Zanetti M, Schottle PB, et al. Spring ligament complex: MR imaging-anatomic correlation and findings in asymptomatic subjects. Radiology 2005;237:242–9.

17. Desai K, Beltran L, Bencardino J, et al. The spring recess of the anterior subtalar joint: depiction on MR images with cadaveric correlation. Accepted for presentation at the 2010 ARRS annual meeting. San Diego (CA), May 2–7, 2010.

18. Oh CS, Won HS, Hur MS, et al. Anatomic variations and MRI of the intermalleolar ligament. Am J Roentgenol 2006;186:943–7.

19. Rosenberg ZS, Cheung Y, Beltran J, et al. Posterior intermalleolar ligament of the ankle: normal anatomy and MR imaging features. Am J Roentgenol 1995; 165:387–90.

20. Buschmann WR, Cheung Y, Jahss MH. Magnetic resonance imaging of anomalous leg muscles: accessory soleus, peroneus quartus and the flexor digitorum longus accessorius. Foot Ankle 1991;12: 109–16.

21. Rosenberg ZS, Bencardino J, Cheung YY, et al. Normal muscle variants of the ankle. Radiology 1997;205(P):645.

22. Cheung YY, Rosenberg ZS, Ramsinghani R, et al. Peroneus quartus muscle: MR imaging features. Radiology 1997;202:745.

23. Cheung YY, Rosenberg ZS, Colon E, et al. MR imaging of the accessory flexor digitorum longus tendon. Skeletal Radiol 1999;28:130–7.

24. Ekstrom JE, Shuman WP, Mack LA. MR imaging of accessory soleus muscle. J Comput Assist Tomogr 1990;14:239–42.

25. Yu JS, Resnick D. MR Imaging of the accessory soleus muscle appearance in six patients and a review of the literature. Skeletal Radiol 1994;23:525–8.

26. Romanus B, Lindahl S, Stener B. Accessory soleus muscle. A clinical and radiographic presentation of eleven cases. J Bone J Surg 1986;68:731–4.

27. Lawson JP. Not so normal variants. Orthop Clin North Am 1990;21:483–95.

28. Miller TT, Staron RB, Feldman F, et al. The symptomatic accessory tarsal navicular bone: assessment with MR imaging. Radiology 1995;195:849–53.

29. Bernaerts A, Vanhoenacker FM, Van de Perre S, et al. Accessory navicular bone: not such a normal variant. Belgian J Radiol 2004;87:250–2.

30. Lovejoy CO, Latimer B, Suwa G, et al. Combining prehension and propulsion: the foot of *Ardipithecus ramidus*. Science 2009;326:72, 72e1–72e8.

31. Le Minor JM. Comparative anatomy and significance of the sesamoid bone of the peroneus longus muscle (os peroneum). J Anat 1987;151:85–99.

32. Mota JM, Rosenberg ZR. Magnetic resonance imaging of the peroneal tendons. Top Magn Reson Imaging 1998;9:273–85.

33. Sobel M, Pavlov H, Geppert MJ, et al. Painful os peroneum syndrome: a spectrum of conditions responsible for plantar lateral foot pain. Foot Ankle Int 1994;15:112–24.

34. Karasick D, Schweitzer ME. The os trigonum syndrome: imaging features. Am J Roentgenol 1996;166:125–9.

35. Lawson JP. Clinically significant radiologic anatomic variants of the skeleton. Am J Roentgenol 1994;163: 249–55.

36. Karasick D. Fractures and dislocations of the foot. Semin Roentgenol 1994;29:152–75.

37. Mellado JM. Accessory ossicles and sesamoid bones of the ankle and foot: imaging findings, clinical significance and differential diagnosis. Eur Radiol 2003;12:L164–77.

38. Bencardino J, Rosenberg ZS, Beltran J, et al. Os sustentaculi: depiction on MR images. Skeletal Radiol 1997;26:505–6.

39. Karasick D, Schweitzer ME. Disorders of the hallux sesamoid complex: MR features. Skeletal Radiol 1998;27:411–8.

40. Taylor J, Sartoris DJ, Huang G, et al. Painful conditions affecting the first metatarsal Sesamoid bones. Radiographics 1993;13:817–30.

41. Edwards ME. The relations of the peroneal tendons to the fibula, calcaneus, and cuboideum. Am J Anat 1928;42:213–53.

42. Rosenberg ZS, Beltran J, Cheung YY, et al. MR features of longitudinal tears of the peroneus brevis tendon. Am J Roentgenol 1997;168:141–7.

43. Saupe N, Mengiardi B, Pfirrmann C, et al. Anatomic variants associated with peroneal tendon disorders: MR imaging findings in volunteers with asymptomatic ankles. Radiology 2007;242:509–17.

44. Thompson FM, Patterson AH. Rupture of the peroneus longus tendon. J Bone Joint Surg Am 1989; 71-A:293–5.

45. Boles MA, Lomasney LM, Demos TC. Enlarged peroneal process with peroneus longus tendon entrapment. Skeletal Radiol 1997;26:313–5.

46. Sarrafian S. Anatomy of the foot and ankle. 2nd edition. Philadelphia: Lippincott; 1993.

47. Pomerantz SJ, Kim TW. Pitfalls and variations in neuro orthopaedic MRI. Cincinnati (OH): MRI-EFI Publications; 1995. 6.1–6.54.

48. Miller TT, Bucchieri JS, Joshi A, et al. Pseudodefect of the talar dome: an anatomic pitfall of ankle MR imaging. Radiology 1997;203:857–8.

49. Delfault EM, Rosenberg ZS. Step off and incongruities at Lisfranc joint in asymptomatic individuals: MR imaging features. Radiology 1998;209:345.

50. Shabshin N, Schweitzer ME, Morrison W. High-signal T2 changes of the bone marrow of the foot and ankle in children: red marrow or traumatic changes? Pediatr Radiol 2006;36:670–6.

51. Laor T, Jaramillo D. MR imaging insights into skeletal maturation: what is normal? Radiology 2009;250:28–38.

52. Zubler V, Mengiardi B, Pfirrmann CW, et al. Bone marrow changes on STIR MR images of asymptomatic feet and ankles. Eur Radiol 2007;17:3066–72.

53. Elias I, Zoga AC, Raikin SM, et al. Incidence and morphologic characteristics of benign calcaneal cystic lesions on MRI. Foot Ankle Int 2007;28: 707–14.

54. Fleming JL 2nd, Dodd L, Helms CA. Prominent vascular remnants in the calcaneus simulating a lesion on MRI of the ankle: findings in 67 patients with cadaveric correlation. Am J Roentgenol 2005; 185:1449–52.

55. Elias I, Zoga AC, Schweitzer ME, et al. A specific bone marrow edema around the foot and ankle following trauma and immobilization therapy: pattern description and potential clinical relevance. Foot Ankle Int 2007;28:463–71.

56. Resnick D, Kransdorf MJ. Bone and joint imaging. 3rd edition. Philadelphia: Elsevier Saunders; 2005. p. 975.

57. Jahss MH. Miscellaneous soft-tissue lesions. In: Jahss MH, editor. Disorders of the foot and ankle: medical and surgical management. 2nd edition. Philadelphia: Saunders Company; 1991. p. 1514–39.

58. Hernandez PA. Clinical aspects of bursae and tendon sheaths of the foot. J Am Podiatr Med Assoc 1991;81:366–72.

59. Hartmann. The tendon sheaths and synovial bursae of the foot. Foot Ankle 1981;1:247–69.

60. Sarrafian SK. Tendon sheaths and bursae. In: Sarrafian SK, editor. Anatomy of the foot and ankle: descriptive, topographic, functional. 2nd edition. Philadelphia: Lippincott; 1993. p. 283–93.

61. Brown RR, Rosenberg ZS, Schweitzer ME. MRI of the medial malleolar bursa. Am J Roentgenol 2005; 184:979–83.

62. Pavlov HP, Heneghan MA, Hersh A. The Haglund syndrome: initial and differential diagnosis. Radiology 1982;144:83–8.

63. Pfirrman CW, Zanetti M, Hodler J. Joint MR imaging: normal variants and pitfalls related to sports injury. Magn Reson Imaging Clin N Am 2003;11:193–205.

64. Lohman M, Kivisaari A, Vehmas T, et al. MR imaging abnormalities of foot and ankle in asymptomatic, physically active individuals. Skeletal Radiol 2001; 30:61–6.

65. Zanetti M, Strehle KL, Zollinger H, et al. Morton neuroma and fluid in the intermetatarsal bursae on MR images of 70 asymptomatic volunteers. Radiology 1997;203:516–20.

66. Bencardino J, Rosenberg ZS, Beltran J, et al. Morton's neuroma: is it always symptomatic? Am J Roentgenol 2000;175:649–53.

Magnetic Resonance Imaging of the Midfoot and Forefoot: Normal Variants and Pitfalls

Conor P. Shortt, MB BCh, MSc, FRCR, FFR RCSI

KEYWORDS

• MRI • Foot • Normal variants • Pitfalls • Artifacts

For the purposes of this discussion the midfoot is defined as that region of the foot between the Chopart joint (talonavicular and calcaeocuboid articulations) and the Lisfranc (tarsometatarsal) joints. The forefoot is defined as that part of the foot distal to the Lisfranc joints. Structures usually seen in their entirety on magnetic resonance (MR) ankle studies, such as the posterior tibialis tendon, are not discussed.

TECHNIQUE

It is important to tailor each MR examination for the specific clinical question and whenever possible to avoid performing a large field of view study that includes both the midfoot and forefoot, as this may result in an unwanted reduction in spatial resolution. The placement of localizing markers by technologists (eg, vitamin E markers) at the symptomatic site should be encouraged, but should be placed on the dorsal aspect of the foot to avoid unwanted artifact.

As with any MR imaging protocol it is usually prudent to perform the most important sequences first, in case the study is terminated prematurely. The most important sequence is usually a fluid sensitive sequence such as a coronal (short axis of foot) fat-saturated T2 spin echo sequence.

Care must be taken with interpretation of abnormalities on certain sequences. For example, on a T1 spin echo sequence, the signal within tendons may be high as a result of magic angle effect (**Fig. 1**) and so be misinterpreted as tendinosis or tear.[1] This pitfall may be avoided by looking at the fluid sensitive sequence performed in the same plane, which shows no increased signal. This phenomenon occurs when tendon or ligament fibers are oriented at 55° to the main magnetic field when using sequences that use a low echo time (TE) (T1 and proton density).

Midfoot

MR of the midfoot is often included in MR of the ankle. If a study is performed specifically for a lesion at the midfoot, the same imaging planes as the ankle are appropriate, including sagittal short tau inversion recovery (STIR) and T1 spin echo, axial (long axis of foot) proton density and fat-saturated T2, and a coronal (short axis of foot) fat-saturated T2. Coronal (short axis of foot) T1 spin echo may also be of value for assessment of osseous abnormalities.

Forefoot

Forefoot MR protocols should include distal tarsal level through to the distal phalanges. A suggested protocol includes sagittal STIR, T1 spin echo, short-axis T2 fat-saturated and T1 spin echo T1, and long-axis T2 fat-saturated sequences.

Department of Radiology, Thomas Jefferson University Hospital, 132 South 10th Street, Room 1091, Philadelphia, PA 19107, USA
E-mail address: conor.shortt@jefferson.edu

Magn Reson Imaging Clin N Am 18 (2010) 707–715
doi:10.1016/j.mric.2010.07.008

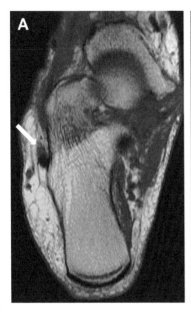
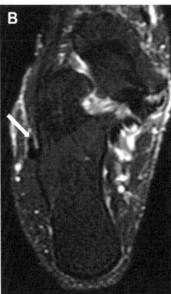

Fig. 1. Magic angle phenomenon. (A) Axial T1 spin echo on a 0.7-Tesla magnet (repetition time [TR] 667, echo time [TE] 10) shows apparent increased signal (magic angle phenomenon) within the midperoneus brevis tendon (*arrow*), located anterior to a normal low signal peroneus longus. (B) Axial fat-saturated T2 spin echo performed at the same level (TR 6800, TE 84) shows normal signal within the peroneus brevis tendon (*arrow*).

Coalitions

Talocalcaneal, calcaneonavicular, talonavicular, and calcaneocuboid coalitions involve at least part of the hindfoot, are readily identified on MR of the ankle, and therefore are not considered in this discussion. Isolated midfoot coalitions usually involve the cuneiforms but are uncommon.

Ossicles and multipartite bones

There are a multitude of potential accessory ossicles and sesamoids in the midfoot and forefoot.[2–4] A complete analysis of each is beyond the scope of this discussion. Nevertheless, some of these ossicles and sesamoids occur frequently and have potential clinical significance.

Accessory or bipartite navicular bones and os peroneii are usually best evaluated on MR of the ankle.

An os intermetatarseum is seen in 1% to 10% of the population.[5,6] It is located dorsally between the medial cuneiform and the base of the first and second metatarsals (**Fig. 2**). It may exist separate from the adjacent bones, articulate with these bones, or fuse with them. Its exact cause is unclear. A true os intermetatarseum can sometimes be symptomatic with associated bone marrow and soft tissue edema.[7–9] A potential pitfall is confusing this entity with an avulsion fracture of the second metatarsal base, which occurs in Lisfranc fractures and dislocations.

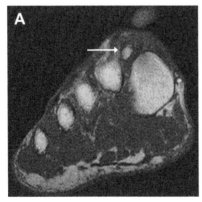
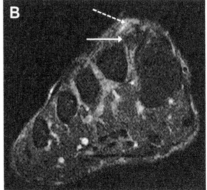

Fig. 2. Os intermetatarseum. (A) Short axial T1 spin echo through the midfoot at metatarsal base level shows an os intermetatarseum located dorsally between the first and second metatarsal (*white arrow*). (B) Short-axis fat-saturated T2 spin echo sequence at the same level shows normal signal in the os without bone edema but dorsal subcutaneous edema (*dashed arrow*) caused by friction.

This pitfall can be avoided by identifying the dorsally positioned os intermetatarseum and lack of injury to the Lisfranc ligaments (see section on Lisfranc injury and **Fig. 3**).

An os supranaviculare has a prevalence of approximately 1%[5] and is located at the dorsal aspect of the talonavicular joint closer to the navicular bone than a similar appearing os supratalare (located anterosuperior to the talar head). It may cause symptoms itself[10,11] but can sometimes be confused with a cortical avulsion of the talar head or navicular bone.

Bipartite bones are occasionally identified at the midfoot, most frequently involving the medial cuneiform (**Fig. 4**). The incidence of this variant is quoted as between 0.3% and 2.4% in the literature.[12,13] The plantar element is usually larger than the dorsal. Knowledge of this entity is important to avoid confusion with fracture of the cuneiform.[14] A pseudoarticulation often intervenes between the 2 elements, which may be a cause for symptoms with degenerative arthropathy, allowing abnormal motion across the joint or sometimes manifesting as fracture through the synchondrosis.[14,15] Features helpful in differentiating between bipartite anatomy and fracture include the bipartite medial cuneiform showing smooth, well-corticated margins and the 2 portions of the bipartite cuneiforms together appearing larger than expected for one normal bone.[14]

Hallux sesamoids

Although sesamoid bones may be seen at other metatarsophalangeal (MTP) joints they are invariably present at the first MTP joint.

The hallux sesamoids (tibial and fibular sesamoids) are an integral part of normal biomechanics of the first MTP joint, assisting in the distribution of forces on flexion of the hallux during walking. They are therefore prone to acute and chronic trauma, leading to a variety of pathologic conditions, including stress response, fracture, degenerative arthropathy at the metatarsosesamoid (MTS) articulation and osteonecrosis. However, there is considerable variation in the size, shape, and number of bones at this site, which may act as confounders in the interpretation of suspected sesamoid abnormality.[2,16]

Overall the frequency of multiple sesamoids at the first MTP joint has been quoted in the literature as ranging from 2.7% to 33.5%[2,17,18]; the presence of a tibial being sesamoid is more common than a fibular. The possibility of bipartite or multipartite morphology at the sesamoids with stress response and/or pseudoarthrosis may present a diagnostic challenge in the setting of suspected fracture, although some features can be used to help differentiate the 2 entities.

Sesamoid fractures usually manifest as a sharp well-demarcated line between the bone fragments, with fluid signal often intervening between. The fragments also usually have the appearance of having once fitted together like a jigsaw puzzle. Bone edema in both fragments at the fracture site and surrounding soft tissue edema are invariably present.

In contrast, bipartite sesamoids with stress response have more rounded sclerotic low T1 signal margins at the interface between the 2 bones, and the 2 bone fragments when added together are larger than the other sesamoid. With stress response, edema of the sesamoids and

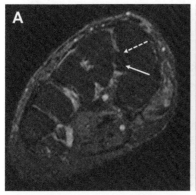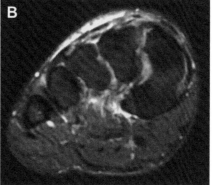

Fig. 3. First Lisfranc ligament disruption. (*A*) Short-axis fat-saturated T2 sequence shows a normal Lisfranc interval between the first and second metatarsal bases with a normal first Lisfranc ligament composed of a dorsal bundle (*dashed arrow*) and a plantar bundle (*solid arrow*). (*B*) Short-axis fat-saturated T2 sequence in a professional athlete after midfoot injury shows soft tissue edema surrounding the first Lisfranc interval and complete disruption of the dorsal and plantar bundles of the ligament.

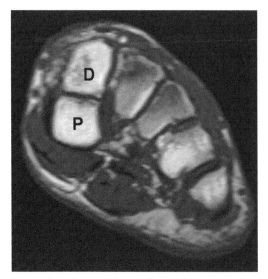

Fig. 4. Bipartite medial cuneiform. Short-axis T1 spin echo through the distal tarsal bones shows a bipartite medial cuneiform with a dorsal (D) and plantar element (P).

periosseous soft tissue are usually not helpful differentiating factors. Fluid signal (high on T2) between the 2 bone fragments may be seen in both pseudoarthrosis and fracture. Clinical history may also be of value in determining the acuteness of symptoms. If any previous imaging is available, this may also be of value in establishing a baseline for comparison.

When disease at the sesamoids is suspected a small field of view centered at this site with sequences in multiple planes is often helpful. In

some circumstances a definitive diagnosis may not be possible initially and correlation with computed tomography for more definitive assessment of a discrete fracture line or follow-up imaging may be needed (**Figs. 5–7**).

Sesamoiditis is a vague term for edema in the sesamoid bones that is nonspecific but often represents a stress response. Edema in the sesamoids is not always due to intrinsic sesamoid abnormality but often reflects degenerative arthropathy at the MTS articulation. To avoid misdiagnosing edema caused by arthropathy and edema caused by other processes (such as stress response, subacute fracture, or avascular necrosis [AVN]), signs of arthropathy should be sought on both sides of the articulation, including subchondral edema, subchondral cyst formation, and osseous productive change.

Sesamoid AVN is likely the last-stage sequela in response to chronic repetitive injury along a spectrum that likely begins with stress response.[19–22] It is manifested by diffuse low-signal T1 marrow replacement with variable but often low signal on T2 fat-saturated sequences. Sometimes areas of T2 hyperintensity can pose a diagnostic dilemma with early AVN or subacute fracture in the differential diagnosis. Signs of chronicity including osteoarthritis manifestations and bursitis suggest AVN as the more likely diagnosis. Features of AVN can also overlap with those of osteoarthritis. However, whereas AVN usually causes diffuse T1 replacement of the affected sesamoid, osteoarthritis usually spares some of the bone, usually the most plantar aspect removed from the MTS joint surface.

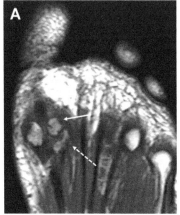
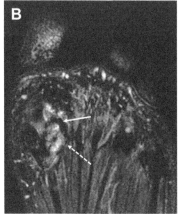

Fig. 5. Bipartite fibular sesamoid with stress response. (*A*) Long-axis T1 spin echo shows a bipartite fibular sesamoid at the first MTP joint with proximal (*dashed arrow*) and distal (*solid arrow*) elements. These 2 fragments, when added together, are almost twice the size of the adjacent tibial sesamoid. Note the sclerotic margins at the junction of the 2 bones. (*B*) Long-axis fat-saturated T2 sequence in the same patient shows edema in both proximal (*dashed arrow*) and distal (*solid arrow*) elements consistent with stress response.

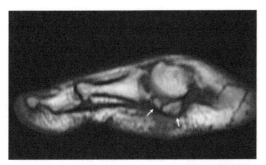

Fig. 6. Bipartite tibial sesamoid. Sagittal T1 sequence showing 2 fragments of a bipartite tibial sesamoid (*arrows*). Note the sclerotic margins at the junction of the 2 bones and their rounded appearance.

Congenital absence of the first MTP sesamoids does exist[23-26] but when this is suspected, the images should be evaluated for evidence of surgery and correlation should be performed with previous imaging and the patient's history.

First MTP Joint

Osteoathritis is common at the first MTP joint and usually not difficult to diagnose, showing the cardinal features of joint space narrowing, subchondral cysts, edema and sclerosis, and osteophyte formation (**Fig. 8**). When a focus of

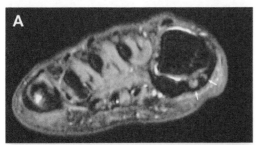

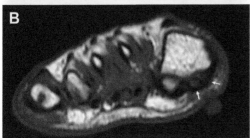

Fig. 7. Tibial sesamoid fracture. (*A*) Short-axis fat-saturated T2 sequence of the foot at metatarsal head level reveals fracture in the sagittal plane of the tibial sesamoid with associated edema in both bone fragments (*arrows*) and adjacent soft tissue edema. (*B*) Short-axis T1 at the some level shows some low-signal T1 replacement in the 2 tibial sesamoid bone fragments (*arrows*) caused by intense edema.

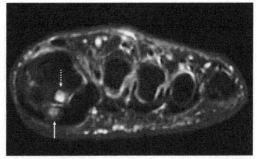

Fig. 8. Metatarsal-sesamoid osteoarthritis. Short-axis fat-saturated T2 weighted sequence shows edema within the tibial sesamoid (*solid arrow*) but reciprocal changes of degenerative arthropathy (osteoarthritis) on the metatarsal side of the metatarsal-sesamoid articulation, manifested by a subchondral cyst in the crista of the metatarsal head (*dashed arrow*).

subchondral signal abnormality is seen it is tempting always to attribute it to osteoarthritis. If the abnormality exists only on 1 side of the joint (eg, in the first metatarsal head), another cause should be diagnosed such as an osteochondral lesion (OCL) or AVN. OCLs although uncommon can be a significant source of pain (**Fig. 9**). A discrete focal cartilage defect may be evident with high-resolution imaging, and/or flattening of the metatarsal head may be seen. This situation can predispose to the subsequent development of degenerative arthropathy.[27] AVN is less common in the absence of surgery but can sometimes be seen in association with an OCL, as is likely in Freiberg infraction of the second metatarsal head. If AVN is a diagnostic consideration, dynamic enhanced imaging may be of value to show areas of ischemia.

Postoperative changes

In the setting of amputation of a toe, it is tempting to call edema in the residual bony stump reactive or postoperative. However, although early weight bearing could cause edema as a result of stress response, any edema at this site, even in the early postoperative period, should be treated as suspicious for infection. Other signs of infection should also be sought such as abnormal enhancement and soft tissue changes such as collections and sinus tracts.

Lisfranc injury

Lisfranc fracture and dislocation are usually not a problem to diagnose on radiographs and MR imaging. Injury to the first Lisfranc ligaments, which provide stability to this articulation, in particular the plantar bundle of this ligament (which extends from the medial cuneiform to the second

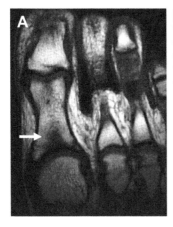
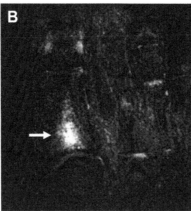

Fig. 9. OCL of the proximal phalanx at the first MTP joint. (*A*) Long-axis T1 sequence of the first MTP joint shows flamelike low signal extending from the subchondral surface of the proximal phalanx (*arrow*) consistent with an OCL. (*B*) This signal abnormality (*arrow*) represents edema as seen on this long-axis fat-saturated T2 sequence. Note the lack of reciprocal changes on the metatarsal head to suggest osteoarthritis.

and third metatarsal bases), may be more subtle, and its diagnosis requires knowledge of the anatomy and patterns of injury. Any edema in or around this ligament should be considered suspicious for significant injury.[28] Secondary signs are particularly useful in raising this suspicion. These signs include bone bruising at the base of the second metatarsal and the inferior aspect of the medial cuneiform, soft tissue edema extending along the second metatarsal shaft, and edema in the first interosseous muscle (see **Fig. 3**).

Intermetatarsal space and the plantar plate

Morton neuroma is perineural fibrosis that occurs around the interdigital nerve as it passes between the metatarsal heads, occurring likely as a result of impingement from repetitive pressure.[29,30] Intermetatarsal bursitis is often associated with a Morton neuroma (**Fig. 10**).

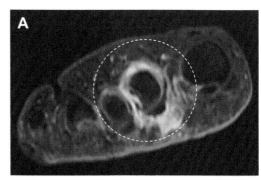
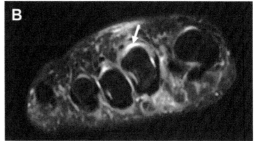

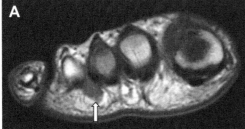
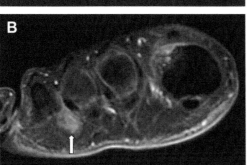

Fig. 10. Morton neuroma. (*A*) T1 short-axis view through the metatarsal heads shows a low-signal mass (*arrow*) protruding in a plantar direction from the third intermetatarsal space. (*B*) T1 fat-saturated short-axis after gadolinium view at the same level reveals enhancement of the Morton neuroma (*arrow*) centered between the metatarsal heads.

Fig. 11. Plantar plate injury. (*A*) Short-axis T1 sequence after gadolinium through the metatarsal heads shows circumferential enhancement (*broken circle*) centered around the second MTP joint in contradistinction to the Morton neuroma seen in **Fig. 13** in which enhancement was centered between the metatarsal heads on the plantar aspect. (*B*) Short-axis fat-saturated T2 sequence reveals high signal effusion in the second MTP joint (*arrow*), another indicator of a capsular or plantar plate injury not a Morton neuroma.

Occasionally, the differential of Morton neuroma versus plantar plate injury arises.

These entities can be differentiated on MR as follows: Morton neuromas are most commonly seen in the second and third intermetatarsal spaces, uncommonly in the fourth, and rarely in the first. They manifest as masses between the metatarsal heads usually on their plantar aspect and are of low signal on T1 and usually enhance. In comparison, the signal abnormality of plantar plate injury is centered about the affected joint, not between the metatarsal heads. This situation can often be substantiated by showing associated enhancement at the plantar aspect of the metatarsal head and often circumferentially around the joint in the setting of capsular injury. The presence of an effusion also supports the diagnosis of capsular and/or plantar plate inury (**Fig. 11**).

Bone marrow edema patterns
Interpretation of the diabetic foot can be challenging as early neuropathic arthropathy may have some overlapping features with infection. In early neuropathic arthropathy diffuse soft tissue and bone marrow edema is common. The bone marrow may also show increased enhancement after contrast. This situation may be misinterpreted as infection. However, this pitfall can be avoided by recognizing that in the absence of ulceration or sinus tracks, infection is unlikely because contiguous spread of infection is generally observed in the diabetic foot.[31-33]

Characteristic patterns of edema are seen in disuse osteopenia, for example as a result of immobilization, and T2 hyperintense foci representing normal red marrow islands are seen in adolescents, both of which should not be confused with other causes of edema (**Figs. 12 and 13**).[34]

Muscle edema and atrophy patterns
The clinical context is important when interpreting muscle edema at the foot. Knowledge of a history of preexisting diabetes, acute injury, chronic pain, or symptoms possibly related to a neurogenic cause is helpful. Diffuse muscle edema and

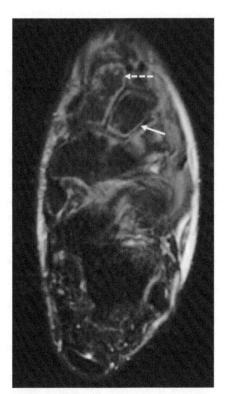

Fig. 12. Immobilization edema. Long-axis fat-saturated T2 sequence through the midfoot shows subcortical edema in the medial (*dashed arrow*) and intermediate (*solid arrow*) cuneiforms typical of immobilization edema caused by disuse osteopenia. This finding is often associated with subcutaneous edema, also seen in this case.

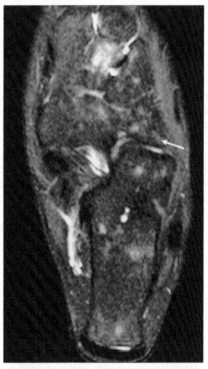

Fig. 13. Hematopoeitic marrow in an adolescent. Long-axis fat-saturated T2 sequence through the midfoot in a 15-year-old girl shows speckled high-signal foci throughout the visualized bones (eg, in the cuboid [*solid arrow*]) representing islands of hematopoietic (red) marrow, commonly seen in adolescents.

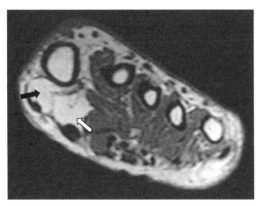

Fig. 14. Medial plantar neuropathy. T1 short-axis sequence through mid metatarsal level shows fatty atrophy of the abductor hallucis (*black arrow*) and flexor hallucis brevis (*white arrow*) muscles caused by medial plantar nerve neuropathy (jogger's foot). Early denervation caused by nerve impingement manifests as edema on fluid sensitive sequences.

atrophy are common in the diabetic foot, and in the absence of other abnormalities usually have little significance.[32] The diagnosis of muscle strains/tears is usually not a problem with findings of edema and an appropriate history. Edema and/or atrophy in specific muscles or muscle groups without such a history should raise suspicion for a neurogenic cause, often nerve impingement (**Fig. 14**).

Muscle variations in the foot

Muscle variations (including accessory muscles, accessory or anomalous slips, and variant attachments) do occur at the mid- and forefoot but, compared with the ankle where these muscles present more often with symptoms, they are frequently asymptomatic. A detailed catalog of these muscle variants is beyond the scope of this discussion, nevertheless the interpreting radiologist should be aware of the potential of accessory muscles to cause symptoms by mass effect and compressive neuropathies. Other texts describe these variants in detail.[35,36]

REFERENCES

1. Mengiardi B, Pfirrmann CW, Schottle PB, et al. Magic angle effect in MR imaging of ankle tendons: influence of foot positioning on prevalence and site in asymptomatic subjects and cadaveric tendons. Eur Radiol 2006;16(10):2197–206.
2. Coskun N, Yuksel M, Cevener M, et al. Incidence of accessory ossicles and sesamoid bones in the feet: a radiographic study of the Turkish subjects. Surg Radiol Anat 2009;31(1):19–24.
3. Mellado JM, Ramos A, Salvado E, et al. Accessory ossicles and sesamoid bones of the ankle and foot: imaging findings, clinical significance and differential diagnosis. Eur Radiol 2003;13(Suppl 6): L164–77.
4. Miller TT. Painful accessory bones of the foot. Semin Musculoskelet Radiol 2002;6(2):153–61.
5. Tsuruta T, Shiokawa Y, Kato A, et al. [Radiological study of the accessory skeletal elements in the foot and ankle (author's transl)]. Nippon Seikeigeka Gakkai Zasshi 1981;55(4):357–70 [in Japanese].
6. Case DT, Ossenberg NS, Burnett SE. Os intermetatarseum: a heritable accessory bone of the human foot. Am J Phys Anthropol 1998;107(2):199–209.
7. Nakasa T, Fukuhara K, Adachi N, et al. Painful os intermetatarseum in athletes: report of four cases and review of the literature. Arch Orthop Trauma Surg 2007;127(4):261–4.
8. Noguchi M, Iwata Y, Miura K, et al. A painful os intermetatarseum in a soccer player: a case report. Foot Ankle Int 2000;21(12):1040–2.
9. Reichmister JP. The painful os intermetatarseum: a brief review and case reports. Clin Orthop Relat Res 1980;153:201–3.
10. Zwelling L, Gunther SF, Hockstein E. Removal of os supranaviculare from a runner's painful foot: a case report. Am J Sports Med 1978;6(1):1–3.
11. Bayramoglu A, Demiryurek D, Firat A, et al. Differential diagnosis in a professional basketball player with foot pain: is it an avulsion fracture or an os supranaviculare? Eklem Hastalik Cerrahisi 2009;20(1): 59–61.
12. Barlow TE. Os cuneiform bipartum. Am J Phys Anthropol 2010;29:95–111.
13. Kjellstrom A. A case study of os cuneiform mediale bipartum from Sigtuna, Sweden. Int J Osteoarchaeol 2010;14:475–80.
14. Elias I, Dheer S, Zoga AC, et al. Magnetic resonance imaging findings in bipartite medial cuneiform – a potential pitfall in diagnosis of midfoot injuries: a case series. J Med Case Reports 2008;2:272.
15. O'Neal ML, Ganey TM, Ogden JA. Fracture of a bipartite medial cuneiform synchondrosis. Foot Ankle Int 1995;16(1):37–40.
16. Frankel JP, Harrington J. Symptomatic bipartite sesamoids. J Foot Surg 1990;29(4):318–23.
17. Kiter E, Akkaya S, Kilic BA, et al. Distribution of the metatarsophalangeal sesamoids in Turkish subjects. J Am Podiatr Med Assoc 2006;96(5):437–41.
18. Aseyo D, Nathan H. Hallux sesamoid bones. Anatomical observations with special reference to osteoarthritis and hallux valgus. Int Orthop 1984; 8(1):67–73.
19. Ozkoc G, Akpinar S, Ozalay M, et al. Hallucal sesamoid osteonecrosis: an overlooked cause of forefoot pain. J Am Podiatr Med Assoc 2005;95 (3):277–80.

20. Toussirot E, Jeunet L, Michel F, et al. Avascular necrosis of the hallucal sesamoids update with reference to two case-reports. Joint Bone Spine 2003;70(4):307–9.

21. Karasick D, Schweitzer ME. Disorders of the hallux sesamoid complex: MR features. Skeletal Radiol 1998;27(8):411–8.

22. Fleischli J, Cheleuitte E. Avascular necrosis of the hallucial sesamoids. J Foot Ankle Surg 1995;34(4): 358–65.

23. Day F, Jones PC, Gilbert CL. Congenital absence of the tibial sesamoid. J Am Podiatr Med Assoc 2002; 92(3):153–4.

24. Le Minor JM. Congenital absence of the lateral metatarso-phalangeal sesamoid bone of the human hallux: a case report. Surg Radiol Anat 1999;21(3): 225–7.

25. Jeng CL, Maurer A, Mizel MS. Congenital absence of the hallux fibular sesamoid: a case report and review of the literature. Foot Ankle Int 1998;19(5): 329–31.

26. Zinsmeister BJ, Edelman R. Congenital absence of the tibial sesamoid: a report of two cases. J Foot Surg 1985;24(4):266–8.

27. Thomas AP, Dwyer NS. Osteochondral defects of the first metatarsal head in adolescence: a stage in the development of hallux rigidus. J Pediatr Orthop 1989;9(2):236–9.

28. Raikin SM, Elias I, Dheer S, et al. Prediction of midfoot instability in the subtle Lisfranc injury. Comparison of magnetic resonance imaging with intraoperative findings. J Bone Joint Surg Am 2009;91(4):892–9.

29. Wu KK. Morton's interdigital neuroma: a clinical review of its etiology, treatment, and results. J Foot Ankle Surg 1996;35(2):112–9.

30. Wu KK. Morton neuroma and metatarsalgia. Curr Opin Rheumatol 2000;12(2):131–42.

31. Gil HC, Morrison WB. MR imaging of diabetic foot infection. Semin Musculoskelet Radiol 2004;8(3): 189–98.

32. Morrison WB, Ledermann HP, Schweitzer ME. MR imaging of the diabetic foot. Magn Reson Imaging Clin N Am 2001;9(3):603–13, xi.

33. Schweitzer ME, Morrison WB. MR imaging of the diabetic foot. Radiol Clin North Am 2004;42(1): 61–71, vi.

34. Weishaupt D, Schweitzer ME. MR imaging of the foot and ankle: patterns of bone marrow signal abnormalities. Eur Radiol 2002;12(2):416–26.

35. Berman RA, Thompson SA, Afiti AK. Compendium of human anatomic variation. Baltimore (MD): Urban & Schwarzenberg; 1988.

36. Bejjani FJ, Jahss MH. Le Double's study of muscle variations of the human body. Part I: Muscle variations of the leg. Foot Ankle 1985;6(3):111–34.

MR Imaging Features of Common Variant Spinal Anatomy

Daniel J. Durand, MD[a,b,*], Thierry A.G.M. Huisman, MD[a,c], John A. Carrino, MD, MPH[a,d]

KEYWORDS

• MR imaging • Spine • Embryology • Normal variant

The spine is one of the most commonly imaged body parts for all age groups, with indications ranging from congenital abnormalities at birth to degenerative pathology toward the end of life. Because of the importance of soft-tissue contrast when imaging the spine, MR imaging has become the most important modality in its evaluation. One of the key challenges in the clinical analysis of spinal MR imaging lies in the wide range of so-called normal variability. The goal of this article is not to provide the reader with an exhaustive atlas detailing the appearance of every known variant. Instead, the authors review the MR appearance of the most important variants and provide a logical and, it is hoped, memorable framework for assimilating this information into practice. To understand why these variations occur, the authors examine the aberrant pathways of embryology, growth, and development that lead to their formation.

Before beginning this task, it is important to remember that the definition of *normal* variant anatomy is itself somewhat arbitrary and vague. For example, normal variants, such as transitional lumbar vertebra, may set the stage for accelerated degenerative arthritis later in life.[1] Similarly, many variants that are normal in isolation can be seen in association with more complex and distinctly pathologic congenital malformations of the spine and other organs. For the purposes of this article, the authors consider normal those variants that do not cause immediate pathology by early adulthood, with the understanding that in the future, as medical knowledge advances, these variants may eventually be considered pathologic and may even be addressed prophylactically.

NORMAL EMBRYOLOGY AND DEVELOPMENT

As a practicing radiologist, it is easy to conceive of the spine as a *fait accompli* and take for granted the miracle by which the majority of this intricate structure is formed within a matter of weeks beginning with a single cell. The spine is a marvel of form and function, providing key mechanical support while protecting its most delicate and essential neural structures. It is not surprising that considerable variability should arise from such complexity.

Formation of the Vertebral Column

The embryologic precursors of the spine appear in the third week of gestation during gastrulation when the primitive streak forms on the bilaminar embryonic disc, heralding the migration of epiblastic cells through the streak to form a new layer of mesodermal cells interspersed between the layers of the bilaminar disc, thus forming the

[a] Russell H. Morgan Department of Radiology and Radiological Science, Johns Hopkins Medical Institutions, 601 North Caroline Street, Baltimore, MD 21287, USA
[b] Department of Johns Hopkins Musculoskeletal Radiology, Johns Hopkins Medical Institutions, 601 North Caroline Street, Room 5165, Baltimore, MD 21287, USA
[c] Division of Pediatric Radiology, Johns Hopkins Medical Institutions, 600 North Wolfe Street, Nelson Basement, B-173, Baltimore, MD 21287-0842, USA
[d] Division of Musculoskeletal Radiology, Johns Hopkins Medical Institutions, 601 North Caroline Street, Room 5165, Baltimore, MD 21287, USA
* Corresponding author. Johns Hopkins Musculoskeletal Radiology, 601 North Caroline Street, Room 5165, Baltimore, MD 21287.
E-mail address: Durand@jhmi.edu

Magn Reson Imaging Clin N Am 18 (2010) 717–726
doi:10.1016/j.mric.2010.09.005

trilaminar embryonic disc (**Fig.** 1A, B).[2] Along the cranial end of the primitive streak is the primitive node. Cells migrating through the node give rise to the prechordal plate and the notochordal process.[3] It is the notochordal process that eventually becomes the notochord, the embryonic structure most directly responsible for vertebral development. The notochord itself consists of a mucoid matrix with sparse polygonal cells and acts as a kind of scaffold upon which mesodermal cells will organize to give rise to the vertebral column.[4]

On either side of the notochord, the mesoderm differentiates into 3 parts, one of which is called the paraxial mesoderm.[3] The paraxial mesoderm forms the somites, also called the primitive segments,

which are masses of bilaterally symmetric regularly spaced cells (see **Fig.** 1C–F). The somites themselves are composed of a sclerotome consisting of cells that will ultimately form the vertebral column, and a dermomyotome consisting of cells that will ultimately form the overlying muscles and skin. Also around this time, the cells along the ectodermal side of the notochord undergo the process of neurulation, whereby the neural plate involutes and fuses to form the neural tube, the precursor of the central nervous system comprising the brain and the spinal cord.[2]

During the fourth week of gestation, the sclerotomes migrate and surround the notochord and the overlying neural tube. Each sclerotome then separates into 2 distinct layers, forming a cranial

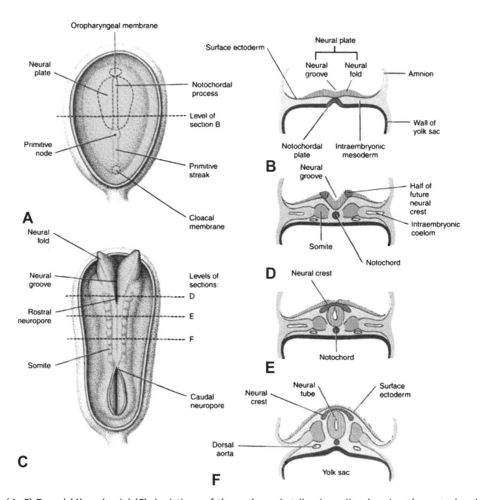

Fig. 1. (*A, B*) Dorsal (*A*) and axial (*B*) depictions of the embryonic trilaminar disc showing the notochordal and neural tube plates before fusion at approximately day 18. (*C*) Dorsal view of the embryo at approximately 22 days showing closure of the neural tube in both directions as well as bilaterally symmetric somites. (D–F) Axial views at different levels of (*C*) show unfused (*D*), partially fused (*E*) and completely fused (*F*) neural tube demonstrating the relationship between the sclerotomes, notochord, neural tube, and neural crest cells at these stages. (*From* Moore KL, Persaud TV, Shiota K. Color atlas of clinical embryology. Philadelphia: Saunders; 1994. p. 210; with permission.)

area of loosely packed cells and a caudal area of densely packed cells (**Fig. 2**). Between these 2 areas is a *cell-free space* that will eventually become the site of the intervertebral disc as some mesenchymal cells later migrate into this space to form the annulus fibrosis, leaving the remnants of the notochord to form the nuclear pulposus.[5] The centrum, which will eventually form the vertebral body, is then formed by the cranial, dense area of one somite fusing with the caudal, loose area of the somite immediately cranial to it. Thus, the formation of a normal vertebral body is the result of an intricate union between portions of 2 adjacent somites.[5] The portions of the sclerotomes that surrounded the neural tube go on to form the neural arches, which form the posterior bony elements of the spinal column.

During the sixth week of gestation, signals from the notochord and neural tube lead to chondrification, which ultimately leads to ossification, at which point the notochord disintegrates.[6] There are 3 main ossification centers within each vertebra, one in the centrum and one on each side of the neural arch (**Fig. 3**A). Complete fusion of the 2 portions of the posterior elements is not complete until 6 years of age; whereas, fusion of the vertebral body with the posterior elements is typically not complete until 5 to 8 years of age.[3] Five additional ossification centers form after birth (see **Fig. 3**B), one for each transverse process, one for the spinous process, and one each for the superior and inferior vertebral body endplates.[3]

Several notable exceptions to the classical segmentation pattern occur at the occipitocervical junction. The cranial portion of the first cervical sclerotome, sometimes called the proatlas, undergoes complex and unique segmentation and contributes to the occipital condyles, the dorsal cranial articular processes of C1, and the tip of the odontoid process.[7] The caudal portion

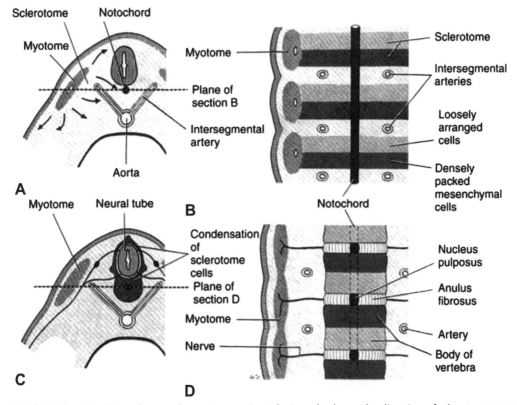

Fig. 2. (*A*) Axial section through an embryo at approximately 4 weeks shows the direction of sclerotome mesenchymal cell migration toward the midline. (*B*) A coronal section at 4 weeks depicting the organization of each sclerotome into a densely packed caudal area and a loosely packed cranial zone. (*C*) Axial section at 5 weeks shows that the sclerotomal mesenchymal cells have now condensed around the notochord and neural tube, where they give rise to the centrum and neural arches, respectively. (*D*) Coronal section at 5 weeks depicting that the caudal end of each sclerotome has fused with the cranial end of the preceding sclerotome to form a series of vertebral bodies. Mesenchymal cells form the annulus fibrosis; whereas, notochord regresses to form the nuclear pulposus at the center of the disc. (*From* Moore KL. The developing human: clinically oriented embryology. 4th edition. Philadelphia: Saunders; 1988. p. 338; with permission.)

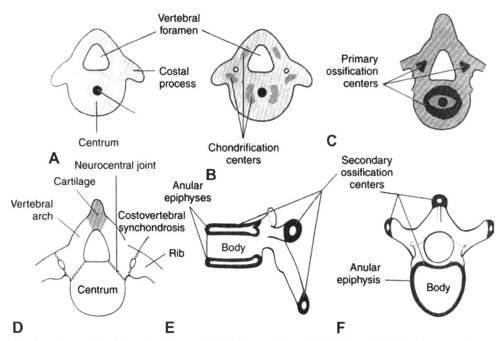

Fig. 3. Various stages of vertebral development. (*A*) Embryo at 5 weeks, similar to **Fig.** 2A and B, showing condensation of mesenchymal cells around the neural tube and notochord. (*B*) Formation of the primary chondrification centers within the embryo at 6 weeks. (*C*) The 3 primary ossification centers within the centrum and bilateral neural arches depicted within a thoracic vertebra at approximately 7 weeks. Although the timing of ossification varies according to level, all vertebrae, except C1 and C2, ossify in this manner. (*D*) Thoracic vertebra at birth with lack of complete fusion of the posterior arch and residual cartilage between the arches and centrum at the neurocentral joints. (*E, F*) Views of a thoracic vertebral body at puberty showing secondary ossification centers. (*From* Moore KL. The developing human: clinically oriented embryology. 4th edition. Philadelphia: Saunders; 1988. p. 338; with permission.)

of the C1 sclerotome forms the anterior and posterior arches of C1 as well as contributing to the odontoid process. The C1 anterior ossification center typically does not ossify until 1 year of age and complete fusion of the anterior with the posterior arches to form the C1 ring is not complete until 7 years of age.[8] The axis is the most complex of all vertebrae and contains 6 ossification centers in utero derived from 2 sclerotomes. Three are derived from the C2 sclerotome, a bilaterally symmetric pair that correspond to the centrum of C1[8] and the apex of the odontoid, which is derived from the proatlas. The odontoid process will fuse with the body of C2 between 3 and 6 years of age, although a remnant of the apophyseal fusion line can persist up to 11 years of age. A secondary ossification center appears cranial to the odontoid process, termed the ossiculum terminale, at 3 years of age and does not fuse until approximately 12 years of age.[8]

The final developmental aspect of the spine to consider is its curvature. The normal curvature of the fetal and newborn spine is kyphotic. The cervical and lumbar lordosis emerge after birth and are thought to be functional in origin: the cervical curvature resulting primarily because of the infant holding his head upright and the lumbar lordosis emerging later in development as the infant/toddler assumes an erect posture.[2]

Formation of the Spinal Cord

Formation of the spinal cord is classically divided into 2 main movements: primary and secondary neurulation. Primary neurulation begins in week 3 when the newly formed notochord induces the adjacent ectoderm to form 2 ridges that fuse to form the neural tube, the structure that will ultimately give rise to the brain and spinal cord. Fusion begins at or near the fourth somite and proceeds in both directions, typically complete by day 26.[9]

The process of secondary neurulation refers to the formation of additional caudal elements of the spinal cord and is further divided into canalization and retrogressive differentiation. During the process of canalization, a group of undifferentiated cells at the caudal end of the neural tube develops cysts or vacuoles that merge with one another and eventually with the central canal of the caudal end of the cord to further elongate the neural tube. Retrogressive differentiation refers to the process whereby the caudal cell mass regresses, eventually leaving only the conus medullaris, ventricular laminalis, and the filum terminal. The process of primary neurulation accounts for structures as caudal as somite 31, or the vertebral level of S2. Vertebral bodies up to S2 are thus derived from the notochord whereas those below S2 derive from the caudal cell mass.[10]

VARIANT ANATOMY
Variants of Formation

Variants of formation, as their name implies, result from the failure of all or part of a vertebral body to form during development. There does not appear to be any single agreed upon mechanism for this failure in development and a broad clinical spectrum may result ranging from entirely occult lesions to debilitating scoliosis. Because this article is devoted to normal variants, the authors examine subtle cases of isolated variation unlikely to have caused any structural or functional consequence, although all can be seen in association with genuinely pathologic variants. It is important to note that these can occur in any combination with the segmentation anomalies listed in the next section, resulting in a wide range of combinatorial variation.

Hemivertebrae (**Fig. 4**) occur when half of a vertebral body does not develop because of complete unilateral failure of one of the bilaterally symmetric embryonic chondrification centers that normally fuse to form the centrum. Incarcerated hemivertebrae, in which the curvature of the spine is unaffected, carry the best prognosis.[2] *Wedge vertebrae* result from hypoplasia of one half of the vertebral body, typically caused by incomplete unilateral failure of one of the ossification centers. Note that wedge vertebrae, by definition, cannot be entirely incarcerated, although the affect on the overall structure of the spine may be mitigated by compensatory changes in shape of the vertebrae above and below. In children, nonsegmented wedge vertebrae have a more benign course in that they have no growth potential; whereas, properly segmented wedge vertebrae may cause a defect that worsens progressively with growth.[2] Hemivertebrae and wedge vertebrae are part of the same spectrum and can be difficult to distinguish from one another. Consider, for example, the result of a nonsegmented hemivertebra fused to an adjacent level. The only true way to tell this apart from a wedge vertebra would the presence of an extra pedicle on the side of the nonsegmented hemivertebra.

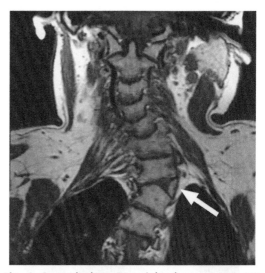

Fig. 4. Coronal plane T1-weighted noncontrast MR image showing a left-sided hemivertebra at T2 with complete segmentation. Note that this anomaly results in considerable levoscoliosis in the upper thoracic and lower cervical spine.

Variants of Segmentation

Variants of segmentation occur when 2 contiguous vertebral bodies fail to separate. As previously stated, this is often seen in combination with formation defects resulting in a wide array of pathology. Segmentation anomalies are thought to result from failure of 2 somites to separate during segmentation. As a result, a growth plate is lost, which limits the growth potential of nonsegmented vertebrae.

Block vertebrae (**Fig. 5**) result from failure of intervertebral disc formation resulting in total fusion of 2 contiguous vertebrae. Note that this results in loss of 2 growth plates: the superior endplate growth center of the lower vertebral body as well as the inferior endplate growth center of the upper vertebral body. As a result, block vertebrae have a lower growth potential. On MR imaging, as with other imaging, they are characterized by the presence of 2 ipsilateral contiguous pedicles without an intervening intervertebral disc. Though rare, block vertebrae occur most often within the cervical spine, with C2 to C3 the most commonly affected level in one recent study.[11] Block vertebrae can be complete or incomplete and may involve fusion of only the anterior or posterior portions of the involved vertebral bodies, which can cause resultant kyphotic and lordotic anomalies of spinal curvature, respectively. *Unilateral bar vertebrae* result from a failure of only part of the intervertebral disc to form, resulting in partial

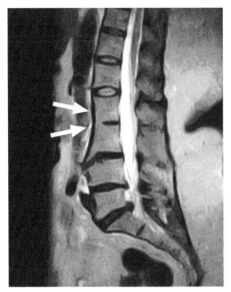

Fig. 5. Sagittal plane, T2-weighted noncontrast image through the lumbar spine showing an incomplete block vertebra at L2 to L3 with incomplete segmentation of the anterior vertebral bodies. Note that this interrupts the normal lumbar lordosis.

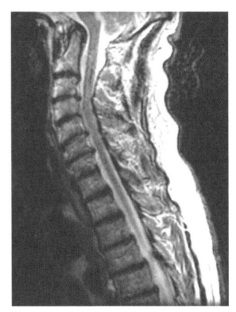

Fig. 6. Sagittal place, T1-weighted noncontrast image showing fusion of the anterior arch of C1 to the occiput.

fusion of the contiguous vertebral bodies. Because the involved portion will lack 2 growth plates as previously detailed, this typically results in asymmetric growth that becomes more apparent as patients mature. Bar vertebrae, therefore, are more likely to represent pathology though it is possible that mild occult cases would fall under the description of a normal variant.

Atlantooccipital fusion (occipitalization of C1) **(Fig. 6)** is similar to a block vertebra fused cervical vertebrae with the exception that the segmentation failure involves the proatlas or the C1 sclerotome[12] The incidence of atlantooccipital fusion is probably less than 0.75%.[13]

Variants of Fusion and Cleft Formation

Os odontoideum **(Fig. 7)** refers to the presence of a rounded ossicle at the location of the cranial most portion of the odontoid process and exists as part of a spectrum of odontoid anomalies ranging from aplasia to hypoplasia to Os odontoideum and Os terminale, which together have been called the Os terminale-Os odontoideum complex.[14] The underlying cause of Os odontoideum remains controversial, with strong arguments offered for both congenital[7] and acquired (ie, posttraumatic) etiologies,[15] or both.[14] Congenital Os odontoideum arises when there is failure of fusion between the two cranial-most ossification centers of the axis, which are derived from C1

and the proatlas, respectively.[7] In some cases, Os odontoideum can be associated with atlantoaxial instability.[16] On imaging, the ununited os may be seen either in the expected location of the dens (orthotopic) or at the base of the

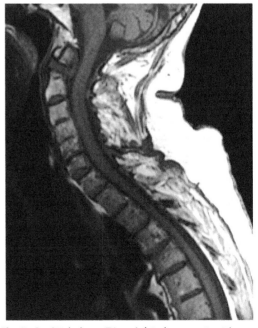

Fig. 7. Sagittal plane, T1-weighted noncontrast image showing nonunion of the body and tip of the odontoid; an *orthotopic* Os odontoideum.

atlantoaxial joint (dystopic).[15] In some cases, the os is fused to the anterior arch of C1.[14] Some investigators consider os terminale or ossiculum terminale [17] to be a normal variant distinct from Os odontoideum in that it results from nonfusion of the secondary ossification center at the cranial end of the odontoid process. Like Os odontoideum, both developmental and posttraumatic etiologies have been ascribed to ossiculum terminale.

Butterfly vertebrae (**Fig. 8**) are characterized by a sagittal midline cleft and are thought to arise from failure of bilaterally symmetric chondrification centers to fuse at the midline and form the centrum, which would normally occur between the third and sixth week of embryonic development.[18] The result is a vertebral body with a short or absent center (the butterfly's body) and 2 larger lateral masses (its wings), which is sometimes accompanied by mild abnormalities in the adjacent vertebral bodies. Butterfly vertebrae can occur in association with a variety of syndromes, but may also rarely be seen in isolation and are most common in the lower thoracic or upper lumbar vertebrae. In some instances a persistent notochord can mimic the appearance of a butterfly vertebra (see *persistent notochord* in a later discussion).[19]

Spina bifida occulta is one of the most common spinal variants and consists of incomplete fusion of the posterior elements, most often in the lower spinal segments.[2] Classically, there is an aberrant patch of dark hair at the surface of the overlying skin thought to be caused by the induction from factors secreted by the neural tube/developing spine. The incidence of spina bifida occulta is on the order of 15% with the lower segments, particularly the sacrum, disproportionately affected.[20] These patients are generally asymptomatic, although associations with subtle neurologic deficits, such as constipation, have been proposed.[21]

There may be additional pathways by which spina bifida occulta can develop, but the most well-accepted pathway is simply failure of fusion of the primary and secondary ossification centers that form the neural arch.[2] Spina bifida occulta is commonly described as lying along the continuum of spinal dysraphisms, lying somewhere between normal and meningocele. However, it is worth noting the important developmental distinction: the neural tube is fully closed in spina bifida occulta. Defects of neural tube closure, such as meningocele and myelomeningocele, result from an earlier and more fundamental defect during the fourth week of gestation.[2]

Spina bifida occult is best demonstrated by CT or radiography, although it also has a characteristic MR imaging appearance. The absent portion of the neural arch is typically replaced by paraspinal fat, which can be challenging to visualize on MR imaging because marrow fat and cellular fat have a similar signal. The key is to look for absence of the rim of signal dropout representing the calcified matrix of the neural arch.

Limbus vertebrae (**Fig. 9**) result from an early intravertebral disc herniation in which case the disc material extends beneath the ring apophysis and prevents fusion with the vertebral body. Limbus vertebrae are most commonly seen in the anterior lumbar spine and, in the setting of acute trauma, can be mistaken for fractures by radiography and CT. On MR imaging, the absence of adjacent bone marrow edema strongly suggests that the abnormality is developmental and not caused by acute fracture.[22]

Miscellaneous Variants

Fatty filum terminale (**Fig. 10**) is fatty replacement of the normally T2 and T1 hypointense filum terminate, a delicate fibrous structure that runs from the conus medullaris to the insert on the back of the first coccygeal vertebra. A recent study found that fatty filum is seen incidentally in approximately 1.3% of patients undergoing MR imaging.[23] The presence of a T1 and T2 hyperintense signal within a filum of uniform caliber measuring 2 mm or less in diameter is pathognomonic for a fatty filum. Fat signal within a filum terminale greater than 2 mm in diameter is technically considered

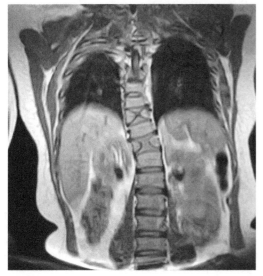

Fig. 8. Coronal plane, T1-weighted noncontrast image showing 2 butterfly vertebra in the lower thoracic spine associated with mild scoliosis.

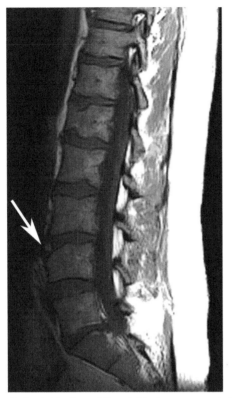

Fig. 9. Sagittal plane, T1-weighted noncontrast MR image of the lumbar spine showing a limbus vertebra at L4. Multiple Schmorl's nodes are also seen within the lumbar spine.

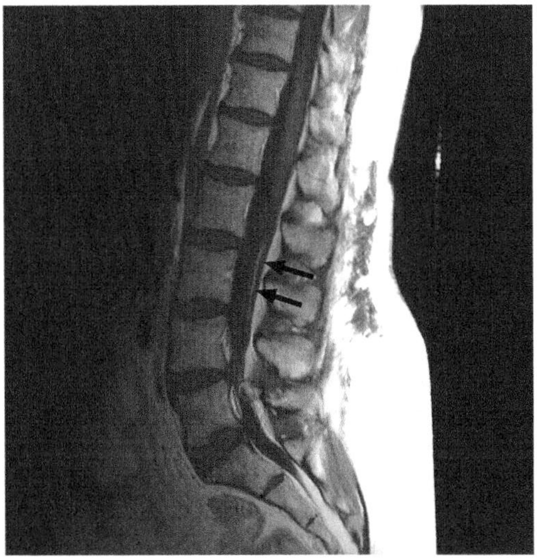

a fibrolipoma of the filum terminale, which carries an increased risk of cord tethering. Fatty filum and fibrolipoma are clearly part of the same spectrum and are thought to result from aberrant differentiation of totipotent cells within the caudal cell mass during secondary neurulation.[24]

Persistent notochord (**Fig. 11**) is a variant in which tracts of remnant notochord tissue are seen within the vertebral bodies, often at multiple levels. During development the notochord essentially functions as the scaffold upon which the mesenchyme organizes to form the somites initially and ultimately the vertebral bodies and intervertebral discs. The notochord itself is composed of polygonal cells suspended in an acellular mucoid matrix,[4] a composition that would presumably make it T2 hyperintense and T1 isointense to hyperintense. During intrauterine development, the intravertebral portion of the notochord is replaced entirely, and the portion at the center of the disc space undergoes mucoid degeneration to form the substance of the nucleus pulposus. The annulus fibrosis, however, is derived from cells of the mesenchymal sclerotomes. Rarely, the intervertebral portion of the notochordal canal can persist well into adulthood, which is thought to result from the persistence of

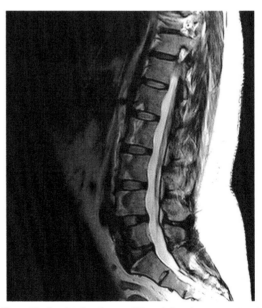

Fig. 11. Sagittal plane, T2-weighted noncontrast image shows a tract of T2 hyperintense tissue interrupting the anterior vertebral bodies at several lumbar levels, representing residual embryonic cartilage of a persistent notochordal canal. There is T2 hypointensity at the interface between the vertebral body and persistent notochordal canal, representing reactive sclerosis.

Fig. 10. Sagittal plane, T1-weighted noncontrast image shows a fatty filum as a linear T1 hyperintense structure coursing from the conus through the lower canal, approximately 2 mm in diameter.

notochordal cells, which, in turn, effect the differentiation of the neighboring mesenchymal cells while they are forming the vertebral body.[4] Specifically, the embryonic cartilage cells never undergo ossification, leaving a column of cartilage running in a tract from the nucleus pulposus at one level to the next. This tract may completely or only partially interrupt the vertebral body and is most commonly seen in the lumbar spine. Because it is composed of cartilage, the canal is T1 hypointense and T2 hyperintense relative to the normal vertebral marrow and may be surrounded by a rim of T1 and T2 hypointensity representing sclerosis of the adjacent normal portion of the vertebra. The remnant notochordal canal may also demonstrate T1 post-contrast enhancement, suggesting that the aberrant cartilage is well vascularized.

Schmorl's nodes (see **Fig. 8**) result from herniation of the intervertebral disk into and through the central portion of the vertebral endplate, most commonly affect the lower thoracic and upper lumbar spine, and are named for G. Schmorl, whose extensive work included descriptions of this lesion.[25] Schmorl's nodes are seen in approximately 30% of the population and are considered an asymptomatic lesion, although they are statistically associated with lumbar disc disease.[26] On MR imaging, they are characterized by extension of the T2 hyperintense disc material into the vertebral body. The margins of the lesion are typically rounded and there is often T1 hypointensity of the adjacent vertebral body representing reactive sclerosis.

Transitional vertebrae are two vertebrae lying at the juncture of 2 different spinal segments (eg, L5, S1) that exhibit characteristic features of the neighboring vertebral class, usually with regard to the shape and fusion pattern of their transverse processes. The most important radiologic implication of transitional vertebrae is that they are easily misnumbered, causing confusion when important findings exist at the transitional level or neighboring levels.[27] For this reason, some centers capture scout views of the spine, including all levels up to the cervical spine even on MR imaging of the lumbosacral region. Because the absolute number of vertebrae is rarely changed, vertebrae are numbered consecutively, counting down from C2. Another convention (the one used at the authors' center) is to define L5 as the vertebral body lying at the level of the iliolumbar ligament and to then number the remainder of the vertebrae based on this landmark.[28] *Sacralization of L5* (**Fig. 12**) occurs when the transverse process of L5 fuses with the sacrum. This fusion can occur unilaterally or bilaterally and may be complete or partial. In some cases,

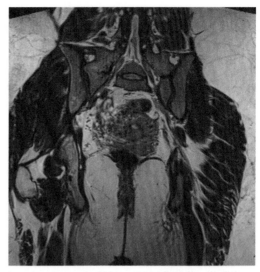

Fig. 12. Coronal plane, T1-weighted noncontrast image shows sacralization of L5 with bilateral pseudarthrosis between the enlarged L5 transverse processes and the sacrum and iliac bones.

a pseudarthrosis may form between the transverse process of a sacralized L5 and the sacrum itself, a finding that may be associated with pain and was first observed on radiography and reported by Bertolotti[29] in 1917. *Lumbarization of S1* occurs when the transverse processes of S1 fails to fuse with the remainder of the sacrum. Though it is unclear whether patients with lumbosacral vertebrae have an increased incidence of degenerative disc disease, it is known that in these patients severe degenerative changes are often found at the disc level immediately above the transitional vertebrae.[1]

SUMMARY

The authors review the MR imaging appearance and developmental basis for the major loci of normal variant anatomy within the spine. In general, these variations occur later in the developmental pathway than pathologic variants, such as neural tube defects. On plain film and radiography, many of these normal variants have an appearance that cannot be reliably distinguished from other pathology, such as traumatic fractures. As a result, it is important to be familiar with the MR imaging appearance of normal variants, because MR imaging is occasionally ordered to distinguish them from acute traumatic injury. When interpreting such studies, it is important to note that for all of the previously mentioned lesions, the absence of marrow edema and adjacent ligamentous injury are important clues that the variation is longstanding and likely normal. The authors are cognizant that this review is not a comprehensive list of every possible anatomic variation within the spine, but hope that this can provide a useful framework whereby readers can continue to assimilate knowledge of additional variants as they encounter them in practice.

REFERENCES

1. Elster AD. Bertolotti's syndrome revisited. Transitional vertebrae of the lumbar spine. Spine 1989;14(12):1373–7.
2. Kaplan KM, Spivak JM, Bendo MD. Embryology of the spine and associated congenital abnormalities. Spine J 2005;5:564–76.
3. Moore K, Persaud TV. The developing human: clinically oriented embryology. 6th edition. Philadelphia: W.B. Saunders Company; 1998.
4. Christopherson LR, Rabin BM, Hallam DK, et al. Persistence of the notochordal canal: mr and plain film appearance. Am J Neuroradiol 1999;20:33–6.
5. O'Rahilly R. Human embryology and teratology. New York: John Wiley & Sons; 1996.
6. Nolting D, Hansen B, Keeling J, et al. Prenatal development of the normal human vertebral corpora in different segments of the spine. Spine 1998;23(21):2265–71.
7. O'Rahilly O, Muller F, Meyer DB. The vertebral column at the end of the embryonic period proper; 2. The occipitocervical junction. J Anat 1983;136:181–95.
8. Lustrin ES, Karakas SP, Ortiz AI, et al. Pediatric cervical spine: normal anatomy, variants, and trauma. Radiographics 2003;23:539–60.
9. Rossi A, Cama A, Piatelli G, et al. Spinal dysraphism: mr imaging rationale. J Neuroradiol 2004;31:3–24.
10. Müller F, O'Rahilly R. The development of the human brain, the closure of the caudal neuropore, and the beginning of secondary neurulation at stage 12. Anat Embryol (Berl) 1987;176:413–30.
11. Leivseth G, Frobin W, Brinchmann P. Congenital block vertebrae are associated with caudally adjacent discs. Clin Biomech (Bristol, Avon) 2005;20:669–74.
12. Richetti ET, States L, Hosalker HS, et al. Radiographic study of the upper cervical spine in the 22q11.2 deletion syndrome. J Bone Joint Surg Am 2004;86:1751–60.
13. Guebert GM, Yochum TR, Rowe LJ. Congenital anomalies and normal skeletal variants. In: Yochum TR, Rowe LJ, editors. Essentials of skeletal radiology. Baltimore (MD): Williams & Wilkins; 1987. p. 107–308.

14. Swischik LE, John SD, Moorthy C. The os terminale - os odontoideum complex. Emerg Radiol 1999;4(2):72–81.
15. Fielding JW, Hensinger RN, Hawkins RJ. Os odontoideum. J Bone Joint Surg Am 1980;62:376–83.
16. Menezes AH. Craniocervical development anatomy and its implications. Childs Nerv Syst 2008;24(10):1109–22.
17. Smoker W. Craniovertebral junction: normal anatomy, craniometry and congenital anomalies. Radiographics 1994;14:255–77.
18. Muller F, O'Rahilly R, Benson DR. The early origin of vertebral anomalies, as illustrated by a "butterfly vertebra." J Anat 1986;149:157–69.
19. Cotten A, Deprez X, Lejeune JP, et al. Persistence of the notochordal canal: plain film. Neuroradiology 1995;37:308–10.
20. Saluja PG. The incidence of spina bifida occulta in a historic and a modern London population. J Anat 1988;158:91–3.
21. Yuan Z, Chen W, Hou A, et al. Constipation is associated with spina bifida occulta in children. Clin Gastroenterol Hepatol 2008;6(12):1348–53.
22. Ghelman B, Freiberger RH. The limbus vertebra: an anterior disc herniation demonstrated by discography. Am J Roentgenol 1976;127:854–5.
23. Iizuka T. Fatty filum terminale on MRI. The Internet Journal of Spine Surgery 2007;3(1) [online].
24. Uchino A, Mori T, Ohno M. Thickened fatty filum terminale: mr imaging. Neuroradiology 1991;33:331–3.
25. Saluja G, Fitzpatrick K, Bruce M, et al. Schmorl's nodes (intravertebral herniations of intervertebral disc tissue) in two historic British populations. J Anat 1986;145:87–96.
26. Williams FN, Manek NJ, Sambrook PN, et al. Schmorl's nodes: common, highly heritable, and related to lumbar disc disease. Arthritis Rheum 2007;57(5):855–60.
27. Hughes RJ, Saifuddin A. Imaging of lumbosacral transitional vertebrae. Clin Radiol 2004;59(11):984–91.
28. Hughes RJ, Saifuddin A. Numbering of lumbosacral transitional vertebrae on MRI: role of the iliolumbar ligaments. Am J Roentgenol 2006;187:W59–65.
29. Bertolotti M. Contributo alla conoscenza dei vizi differenzazione regionale del rachide con speciale riguardo all assimilazione sacrale della V. lombare. Radiol Med 1917;4:113–44 [in Italian].

Bone Marrow

Darra T. Murphy, MB BCh BAO, MRCPI, FFR (RCSI)[a,b,*],
Michael R. Moynagh, MB BCh BAO, MRSC[a],
Stephen J. Eustace, MB BCh BAO, MRCPI, FRCR, FFR (RSCI)[a,b],
Eoin C. Kavanagh, MB BCh BAO, MRCPI, FFR (RSCI)[a]

KEYWORDS

• MR imaging • Bone marrow • Normal variants • Pitfalls

BONE MARROW: CHALLENGES FOR THE RADIOLOGIST

Far from being inert, the bone marrow is a dynamic organ. While composed primarily of water, protein (within cells), and fat, the relative amounts of each are variable not only from person to person depending on their physiologic requirements for the oxygen carrying capacities of hemoglobin but also in the same person over time. As one passes from infancy through childhood and into adulthood, the make-up of bone marrow changes. Just as there are normal variants in every aspect of anatomy, there are normal variants in bone marrow. However, the bone marrow is not immune to disease processes that alter its constituents and often replace them. Radiologists should understand the normal progression of the appearances of bone marrow as one ages, recognize normal variants and normal patterns, and then identify pathologic processes that are manifested by certain disease processes. Although the detection of bone marrow abnormalities is vital for early detection and treatment of disease, false-positive reports of marrow abnormalities can lead to unwanted procedures and the risk of unnecessary treatments. This article explains bone marrow contents and the normal progression of bone marrow changes as they occur throughout the aging process, and provides examples of pitfalls and variants that may simulate disease.

Much has been written in the literature regarding the pathologic changes in bone marrow with disease. Metastatic lesions in bone are approximately 30 times more common than primary bone tumors. The ability to detect these lesions has changed dramatically since the early 1970s when Damadian, Lauterbur and Mansfield began experimenting with magnetic resonance (MR) imaging. The increase in levels of water-bound proteins in metastatic deposits cause these lesions to exhibit signal characteristics that are different from the normal surrounding marrow. However, these lesions are often discrete foci of abnormal signal intensity and are therefore not difficult to detect on T1-weighted sequences, especially against the background high signal intensity of yellow marrow in adults and older children.

Far more challenging to the novice radiologist is the diffuse replacement of marrow in which the signal characteristics of the entire visualized marrow compartment are abnormal or there are symmetric changes. These abnormalities or changes can occur in physiologic and pathologic states, including in smokers, in people living at altitude, and in those with hematologic malignancies, and often as a result of therapeutic effects, including chemotherapeutic and radiotherapeutic effects. Challenges also arise in the pediatric population because of the highly cellular content of their bone marrow. Isolated marrow lesions can appear similar to red marrow on T1-weighted images, and diffuse marrow infiltration can be difficult to distinguish from diffuse hematopoietic marrow, particularly in the acute leukemias.

In these populations, other MR imaging sequences, such as dynamic contrast enhancement and quantitative serial assessments of the fat fraction of bone marrow, are often used to distinguish normal from abnormal bone marrow.

Disclosures: The authors have nothing to disclose.
[a] Department of Radiology, Mater Misericordiae University Hospital, Eccles Street, Dublin 7, Ireland
[b] Department of Radiology, Cappagh National Orthopaedic Hospital, Finglas, Dublin 11, Ireland
* Corresponding author. Department of Radiology, Mater Misericordiae University Hospital, Eccles Street, Dublin 7, Ireland.
E-mail address: darramurphy@me.com

Magn Reson Imaging Clin N Am 18 (2010) 727–735
doi:10.1016/j.mric.2010.07.003

BONE MARROW CONTENTS AND PHYSIOLOGY

From an imaging point of view, the main constituents of the medullary cavity of bone are osseous matrix and bone marrow, of which the latter is divided into red and yellow marrow. Osseous matrix is the cancellous bone that provides the architectural structure for the red and yellow marrow components. It is too simplistic to think of red marrow as being simply made up of cells and yellow marrow as being simply made up of fat; in reality it is more complex, with relative amounts of both present in all marrow (**Fig. 1**).

Bone marrow is made up of fat, water, and protein. The relative amounts of these components vary. In infants and children, red marrow is made up of approximately 40% fat, 40% water, and 20% protein. As one gets older, the relative amount of the fatty elements increase, and by the age of 70 years, red marrow consists of approximately 60% fat, 30% water, and 10% protein. This approximates the relative amounts of the contents of the yellow marrow, which is approximately 80% fat, 15% water, and 5% protein, irrespective of age.

Approximately 95% of yellow marrow is composed of adipocytes, and under the influence of a magnetic field and magnetic gradients, the protons within adipose cells behave differently from those within water; hence the difference in signal intensity.[1]

BONE MARROW SIGNAL INTENSITY

In newborns and infants, red marrow contains little if any fat, having very low signal intensity on both T1- and T2-weighted sequences. This signal is often equal to or lower than that of the adjacent muscle (**Fig. 2**). As the skeleton matures it contains an increasing amount of fat, which leads to increased signal intensity on both T1- and T2-weighted images (**Fig. 3**). On T1-weighted sequences of the lumbar spine in adults, for example, a useful internal reference is that the signal intensity of normal marrow is higher than the signal intensity of the adjacent intervertebral disk.[2] In general, the signal intensity of red marrow is usually higher than that of muscle on T1-weighted images. The exact signal intensity depends on several factors including the cellularity, lipid content, water content, surrounding trabecular bone, iron content of marrow and hematologic components contained within it, and of course the imaging sequence chosen.

On T2-weighted imaging, red marrow also tends be slightly brighter than muscle; however, the signal intensity can approximate that of fatty marrow, hence the need to perform T1-weighted imaging in which the contrast between the two is more pronounced. Fatty marrow, which as discussed contains approximately 95% adipocytes, tends to follow subcutaneous fat signal on both T1- and T2-weighted sequences, due to the short T1 relaxation times (spin-lattice relaxation times) and long T2 relaxation times (spin-spin relaxation times) of the fat protons within the hydrophobic groups contained in relatively heavy molecules.

Bone marrow abnormalities are clearly seen on short-tau inversion recovery (STIR) sequences, which are extensively used in the evaluation of bone marrow and its lesions. Normal fatty marrow has low signal intensity; however, the signal intensity of red marrow is intermediate, similar to that of muscle. STIR sequences are of great value in the evaluation of bone marrow pathologic conditions because of their increased detection of focal lesions in red and yellow marrow, and because they provide reduced motion artefact with fast imaging times.

Trabecular bone has little inherent signal because of its relatively low proton content, but contributes to T2 shortening because of the production of local magnetic field gradients. This effect of trabecular bone becomes even more

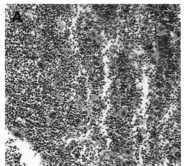
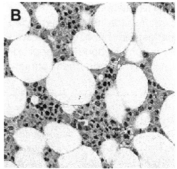

Fig. 1. Histologic specimens of bone marrow demonstrating highly cellular marrow (*A*) and fatty marrow (*B*) (hematoxylin and eosin, original magnification ×200).

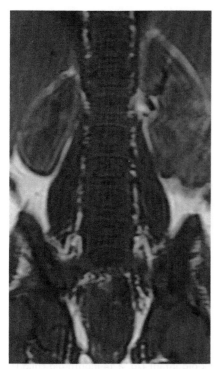

Fig. 2. Coronal T1-weighted spin-echo MR image of the lumbar spine in a 3-month-old infant. The vertebral bodies have lower signal intensity than the intervertebral disks and similar signal intensity as the adjacent muscle, both of which are normal appearances for an infant younger than 6 months.

relevant when gradient echo imaging techniques are used because the magnetic field inhomogeneities are not rephased, leading to decreased signal particularly in the epiphyses and the metaphyses and in the presence of hematopoietic marrow.[3]

Advanced imaging techniques such as MR spectroscopy, chemical shift imaging, diffusion imaging, and dynamic contrast-enhanced imaging are of value in assessing pathologic marrow, although it is important to recognize the normal appearances of marrow on these sequences. In adults, for example, newer studies attempting to show differentiation between benign and malignant causes of vertebral body compression fractures using diffusion-weighted imaging have been performed and discussed in recent literature.[4]

Dynamic contrast-enhanced imaging can be useful in the evaluation of pathologic marrow in children. In children, marrow enhancement may be marked in the developing spine because of increased blood flow, prominent marrow cellularity, and prominent extravascular space that allows pooling of contrast. A potential pitfall in this group is to diagnose a diffuse marrow abnormality in a child solely based on the postcontrast imaging findings of the spinal marrow.

It is not uncommon to see a heterogeneous pattern on T1-weighted images, which may be in the form of high or low signal intensity areas. Heterogeneous marrow conversion can lead to focal fatty involution and therefore focal high signal areas, which are no cause for concern. Difficulty in interpretation arises in cases in which there are focal areas of low signal intensity, and whether to interpret these areas as pathologic or physiologic is of utmost clinical relevance.

Multiple metastatic lesions should not be confused with foci of red marrow that exhibit feathery margins, which interdigitate with fatty marrow and typically show symmetric distribution. Marrow metastases, on the other hand, tend to be more sharply defined and rounded.[5] It is important in these cases to consider the context of the examination and the location, pattern, and distribution of the low signal intensity areas. Also, it is important to note that subepiphyseal rests of red marrow can often be seen in the proximal femora and humeri of normal adult subjects (Fig. 4).

BONE MARROW CONVERSION

Bone marrow conversion is a process that occurs under normal physiologic conditions as one ages. Two sequences of marrow conversion are described.

First, there is the distal to proximal conversion. Conversion occurs initially in the phalanges of the distal extremities even before birth,[6] progressing more proximally throughout the appendicular skeleton in the first and second decades of life.

The second sequence is in the long bones, where marrow conversion begins in the diaphysis of the long bones and progresses to the metaphysis. This progression occurs more rapidly in a distal than in a proximal direction. Infant bones are of low signal intensity on T1-weighted images because of the almost exclusive presence of red marrow. Once the epiphyses ossify, fatty marrow appears within them and therefore the signal intensity changes accordingly (Fig. 5). Any residual low or intermediate signal intensity seen in the epiphyses on T1-weighted sequences after 6 months postossification should be considered abnormal.[7]

In children younger than 10 years, yellow marrow predominates in the diaphyses and metaphyses of all long bones of both upper and lower limbs (Fig. 6) as well as the cranial bones. There can be quite marked heterogeneity of marrow signal in the peripheries where both diffusely heterogeneous and more focal areas of decreased marrow signal can be seen on T1-weighted images, with corresponding high signal on T2-weighted and STIR sequences. In a particular

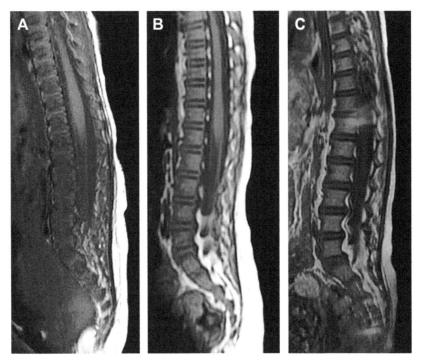

Fig. 3. Sagittal T1-weighted spin-echo MR images from a 3-week-old infant (*A*), a 14-month-old child (*B*), and a 3-year-old child (*C*) show the progression of marrow changes in the axial skeleton in the first few years of life. In the infant, the marrow signal is darker than the signal from adjacent intervertebral disks, a finding that progressively changes as the axial skeleton matures.

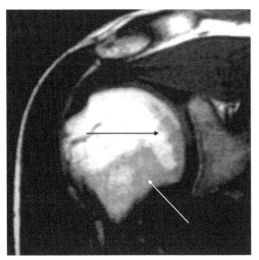

Fig. 4. Coronal T1-weighted spin-echo image of a 32-year-old man shows red marrow rests in the metaphyseal (*white arrow*) and subepiphyseal (*black arrow*) regions. This finding is a normal one in the proximal humerus and a less common one in the proximal femur.

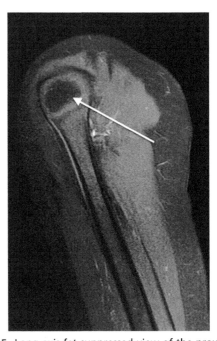

Fig. 5. Long-axis fat-suppressed view of the proximal humerus in a 4-year-old boy. There is low signal intensity in the epiphysis representing suppressed fat signal (*arrow*), as would be expected within 6 months of ossification of the epiphysis.

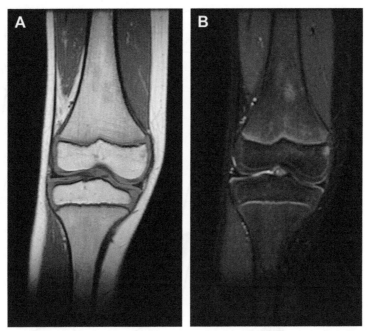

Fig. 6. Coronal T1-weighted spin-echo (*A*) and STIR (*B*) MR images of a knee in a 7-year-old boy show persistent patchy hematogenous marrow in the distal femoral metaphysis, a normal finding in this age group.

study,[8] these changes were seen in 63% of symptomatic and 57% of asymptomatic children. The findings were frequent and bilateral, were thought to represent normal variation of the maturing skeleton, and were not to be interpreted as a sign of pathologic conditions. Similar findings have been described in MR imaging of the foot and ankle[9] as well as the wrist,[10] where age-related changes in signal intensity were seen on fluid-sensitive sequences and were not associated with symptoms of any pathologic condition. The proposed explanation is normal bone remodeling or decreasing hematopoietic marrow, and should not be confused with pathologic bone marrow edema. In these studies, the frequency and intensity of these signal changes decreased with age and with a distal to proximal pattern of resolution.

In the second decade, long bones consist almost entirely of yellow marrow, with red marrow rests remaining in the metaphyses of the humerus and femur (**Figs. 7** and **8**). Toward the end of the second decade, this pattern becomes less prominent (**Fig. 9**) and the adult pattern of yellow marrow distribution is established by the age of 25 years.[11] At this age, red marrow can still be found in the metaphyses of the humerus and femur as well as in the sternum, the ribs, and the axial skeleton.

In early adulthood, when red marrow predominates in the axial skeleton, it is not uncommon to see prominence of fat surrounding the basivertebral veins (**Fig. 10**). In adulthood, marrow conversion from red to yellow occurs more slowly, and indeed the percentage of red marrow persisting in the vertebrae and sternum remains at 50% at the age of 70 years.

A commonly seen pattern is that of hematopoietic marrow hyperplasia, a deviation from the conventional adult pattern of marrow distribution, whereby low to intermediate grade signal intensity is seen on T1-weighted images in the distal femoral metaphyses in patients older than 25 years.[12] This finding is usually an incidental one performed on routine knee MR imaging, with a prevalence varying between 1% and 35% of the population. The finding is usually bilateral, with an increased incidence seen in women. Hematopoietic marrow hyperplasia is also common in athletes, particularly long-distance runners,[13] and heavy smokers (**Fig. 11**).[14] In the latter group, there was also a trend toward seeing this pattern in obese women and people younger than 39 years.

Fatty transformation of marrow can be seen in patients undergoing chemotherapy, and several drugs used in patients with cancer can cause side effects in the immature skeleton, some of which can be misdiagnosed as neoplastic involvement on MR imaging.[15]

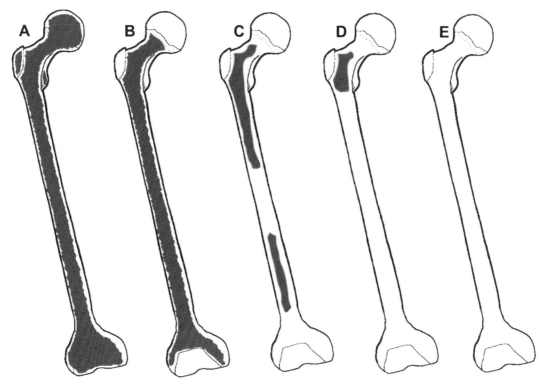

Fig. 7. Red marrow distribution and marrow conversion during infancy (*A*), early childhood (*B*), second decade (*C*), early adulthood (*D*), and adulthood (*E*).

Several articles have described the changes in bone marrow signal postradiotherapy[16,17] on both T1- and T2-weighted images where there is accelerated conversion from red to yellow marrow. Changes are seen as early as several days and persist for years, although they are usually permanent (**Fig. 12**). Usual locations include the thoracic and lumbar spine after

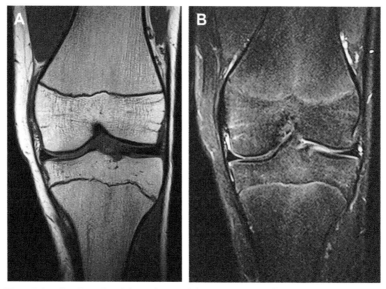

Fig. 8. Coronal T1-weighted spin-echo (*A*) and STIR (*B*) MR images of the knee in a 17-year-old boy show complete absence of any red marrow in the metaphysis by this age. However, prominent hematogenous marrow in the metaphyses can be seen until the end of the second decade.

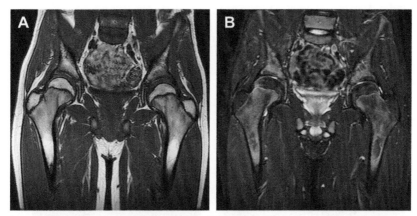

Fig. 9. Coronal T1-weighted spin-echo MR image (*A*) of the pelvis of a 12-year-old boy shows that the femoral metaphyses have an intermediate signal intensity, which is higher than that of muscle and lower than those of the femoral epiphyses and greater trochanters (epiphyseal equivalents), which contain fatty marrow. The corresponding STIR image (*B*) shows appropriate loss of signal in the epiphyses with intermediate signal in the metaphyses, which is lower than that of the intervertebral disk.

radiotherapy for various disorders, including prostate carcinoma, Hodgkin disease, seminoma,[18] and cervical carcinoma,[19] as well as after neoadjuvant therapy for rectal carcinoma.

BONE MARROW RECONVERSION

Marrow reconversion occurs when yellow marrow reconverts to red marrow in response to any increased functional demand for oxygen

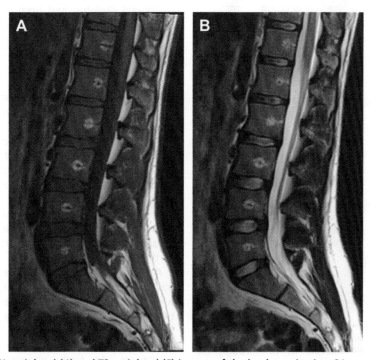

Fig. 10. Sagittal T1-weighted (*A*) and T2-weighted (*B*) images of the lumbar spine in a 21-year-old male patient, which shows high signal corresponding to fat around the basivertebral vein on both sequences, a normal finding not to be confused with that of pathologic condition. The marrow signal is otherwise normal, representing predominantly red marrow in the axial skeleton of this young adult.

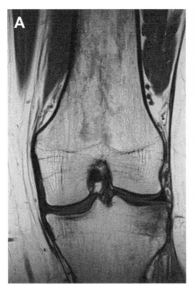 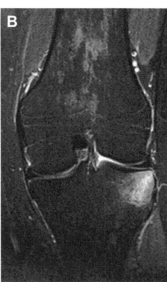

Fig. 11. Coronal T1-weighted spin-echo MR image (*A*) of a 31-year-old woman who sustained an injury to the lateral tibial plateau. Patchy areas of focal and confluent decreased signal were also noted in the diametaphyseal region of the distal femur, with increased signal on the corresponding STIR image (*B*). This patient was a heavy smoker of more than one packet of cigarettes per day, and these findings represent hematopoietic marrow hyperplasia.

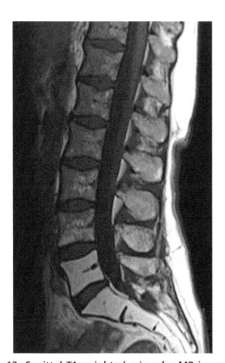

Fig. 12. Sagittal T1-weighted spin-echo MR image in a 59-year-old woman with multiple myeloma. There is patchy abnormal marrow at L1 through L4; however, there is complete fatty replacement at the L5 and sacrum. On further questioning, the patient had received radiation therapy to the pelvis 20 years earlier for the treatment of carcinoma of the cervix.

(or hemoglobin). Reconversion occurs in the reverse order, that is, from the central to the peripheral skeleton and from the metaphysis of long bones to the diaphysis, and is caused by physiologic, pathologic, and iatrogenic stresses. The physiologic stresses can include endurance training,[20] menstruation, and altitude. The pathologic stresses include anemia (except aplastic anemia), chronic obstructive pulmonary disease, anorexia nervosa, and any marrow replacement disorder.

An example of an iatrogenic stress causing bone marrow reconversion is the condition that develops after treatment with certain drugs, particularly granulocyte colony-stimulating factor, in children[21,22] and adults.[23] These changes should not be confused with tumor recurrence. In general, the extent of the reconversion depends on the severity and duration of the insult.

A distinctive pattern of bone marrow edema has been described in the foot and ankle after a variety of weight-bearing and non–weight-bearing immobilization therapies.[24] The pattern has a consistent appearance on MR images and does not seem to be related to clinical symptoms. As such, changes in therapy or further imaging studies are not thought to be necessary on the basis of these MR imaging findings alone.

KEY POINTS: BONE MARROW IMAGING

- T1-weighted turbo spin-echo and STIR MR imaging remains the mainstay of bone marrow evaluation. Other sequences also play a supporting role, most notably diffusion-weighted imaging, MR spectroscopy, and gadolinium-enhanced imaging.
- Bone marrow conversion progresses from distal to proximal in the appendicular skeleton and from diaphysis to metaphysis in the long bones. The epiphysis, except for occasional subepiphyseal rests, should contain only yellow marrow.
- Hematopoietic marrow hyperplasia can give rise to red marrow in the metaphyses of long bones in long-distance runners, heavy smokers, and in persons who are obese.
- Biopsy is necessary in unclear cases in which abnormal bone marrow is identified on MR imaging and cannot be differentiated from normal red marrow.

REFERENCES

1. Burdiles A, Babyn PS. Pediatric bone marrow MR imaging. Magn Reson Imaging Clin N Am 2009; 17(3):391–409, v.
2. Carroll KW, Feller JF, Tirman PF. Useful internal standards for distinguishing infiltrative marrow pathology from hematopoietic marrow at MRI. J Magn Reson Imaging 1997;7(2):394–8.
3. Sebag GH, Moore SG. Effect of trabecular bone on the appearance of marrow in gradient-echo imaging of the appendicular skeleton. Radiology 1990;174 (3 Pt 1):855–9.
4. Biffar A, Dietrich O, Sourbron S, et al. Diffusion and perfusion imaging of bone marrow. Eur J Radiol 2010. [Epub ahead of print].
5. Hwang S, Panicek DM. Magnetic resonance imaging of bone marrow in oncology, Part 1. Skeletal Radiol 2007;36(10):913–20.
6. Emery JL, Follett GF. Regression of bone-marrow haemopoiesis from the terminal digits in the foetus and infant. Br J Haematol 1964;10:485–9.
7. Taccone A, Oddone M, Occhi M, et al. MRI "roadmap" of normal age-related bone marrow. I. Cranial bone and spine. Pediatr Radiol 1995;25 (8):588–95.
8. Pal CR, Tasker AD, Ostlere SJ, et al. Heterogeneous signal in bone marrow on MRI of children's feet: a normal finding? Skeletal Radiol 1999;28(5):274–8.
9. Shabshin N, Schweitzer ME, Morrison WB, et al. High-signal T2 changes of the bone marrow of the foot and ankle in children: red marrow or traumatic changes? Pediatr Radiol 2006;36(7):670–6.
10. Shabshin N, Schweitzer ME. Age dependent T2 changes of bone marrow in pediatric wrist MRI. Skeletal Radiol 2009;38(12):1163–8.
11. Vogler JB 3rd, Murphy WA. Bone marrow imaging. Radiology 1988;168(3):679–93.
12. Deutsch AL, Mink JH, Rosenfelt FP, et al. Incidental detection of hematopoietic hyperplasia on routine knee MR imaging. AJR Am J Roentgenol 1989; 152(2):333–6.
13. Shellock FG, Morris E, Deutsch AL, et al. Hematopoietic bone marrow hyperplasia: high prevalence on MR images of the knee in asymptomatic marathon runners. AJR Am J Roentgenol 1992;158(2):335–8.
14. Poulton TB, Murphy WD, Duerk JL, et al. Bone marrow reconversion in adults who are smokers: MR imaging findings. AJR Am J Roentgenol 1993; 161(6):1217–21.
15. Hwang S, Panicek DM. Magnetic resonance imaging of bone marrow in oncology, Part 2. Skeletal Radiol 2007;36(11):1017–27.
16. Remedios PA, Colletti PM, Raval JK, et al. Magnetic resonance imaging of bone after radiation. Magn Reson Imaging 1988;6(3):301–4.
17. Yankelevitz DF, Henschke CI, Knapp PH, et al. Effect of radiation therapy on thoracic and lumbar bone marrow: evaluation with MR imaging. AJR Am J Roentgenol 1991;157(1):87–92.
18. Stevens SK, Moore SG, Kaplan ID. Early and late bone-marrow changes after irradiation: MR evaluation. AJR Am J Roentgenol 1990;154(4):745–50.
19. Blomlie V, Rofstad EK, Skjonsberg A, et al. Female pelvic bone marrow: serial MR imaging before, during, and after radiation therapy. Radiology 1995;194(2):537–43.
20. Caldemeyer KS, Smith RR, Harris A, et al. Hematopoietic bone marrow hyperplasia: correlation of spinal MR findings, hematologic parameters, and bone mineral density in endurance athletes. Radiology 1996;198(2):503–8.
21. Fletcher BD, Wall JE, Hanna SL. Effect of hematopoietic growth factors on MR images of bone marrow in children undergoing chemotherapy. Radiology 1993;189(3):745–51.
22. Ryan SP, Weinberger E, White KS, et al. MR imaging of bone marrow in children with osteosarcoma: effect of granulocyte colony-stimulating factor. AJR Am J Roentgenol 1995;165(4):915–20.
23. Hartman RP, Sundaram M, Okuno SH, et al. Effect of granulocyte-stimulating factors on marrow of adult patients with musculoskeletal malignancies: incidence and MRI findings. AJR Am J Roentgenol 2004;183(3):645–53.
24. Elias I, Zoga AC, Schweitzer ME, et al. A specific bone marrow edema around the foot and ankle following trauma and immobilization therapy: pattern description and potential clinical relevance. Foot Ankle Int 2007;28(4):463–71.

Index

Note: Page numbers of article titles are in **boldface** type.

Magn Reson Imaging Clin N Am 18 (2010) 737–739
doi:10.1016/S1064-9689(10)00098-X
1064-9689/10/$ – see front matter © 2010 Elsevier Inc. All rights reserved.

mri.theclinics.com

United States Postal Service

Statement of Ownership, Management, and Circulation
(All Periodicals Publications Except Requestor Publications)

1. Publication Title	2. Publication Number	3. Filing Date
Magnetic Resonance Imaging Clinics of North America	0 1 1 - 9 0 0 9	9/15/10

4. Issue Frequency	5. Number of Issues Published Annually	6. Annual Subscription Price
Feb, May, Aug, Nov	4	$309.00

7. Complete Mailing Address of Known Office of Publication (Not printer) (Street, city, county, state, and ZIP+4®)

Elsevier Inc.
360 Park Avenue South
New York, NY 10010-1710

Contact Person
Stephen Bushing
Telephone (Include area code)
215-239-3688

8. Complete Mailing Address of Headquarters or General Business Office of Publisher (Not printer)

Elsevier Inc., 360 Park Avenue South, New York, NY 10010-1710

9. Full Names and Complete Mailing Addresses of Publisher, Editor, and Managing Editor (Do not leave blank)

Publisher (Name and complete mailing address)

Kim Murphy, Elsevier, Inc., 1600 John F. Kennedy Blvd. Suite 1800, Philadelphia, PA 19103-2899

Editor (Name and complete mailing address)

Joanne Husovski, Elsevier, Inc., 1600 John F. Kennedy Blvd. Suite 1800, Philadelphia, PA 19103-2899

Managing Editor (Name and complete mailing address)

Catherine Bewick, Elsevier, Inc., 1600 John F. Kennedy Blvd. Suite 1800, Philadelphia, PA 19103-2899

10. Owner (Do not leave blank. If the publication is owned by a corporation, give the name and address of the corporation immediately followed by the names and addresses of all stockholders owning or holding 1 percent or more of the total amount of stock. If not owned by a corporation, give the names and addresses of the individual owners. If owned by a partnership or other unincorporated firm, give its name and address as well as those of each individual owner. If the publication is published by a nonprofit organization, give its name and address.)

Full Name	Complete Mailing Address
Wholly owned subsidiary of	4520 East-West Highway
Reed/Elsevier, US holdings	Bethesda, MD 20814

11. Known Bondholders, Mortgagees, and Other Security Holders Owning or Holding 1 Percent or More of Total Amount of Bonds, Mortgages, or Other Securities. If none, check box ▸ ☐ None

Full Name	Complete Mailing Address
N/A	

12. Tax Status (For completion by nonprofit organizations authorized to mail at nonprofit rates) (Check one)
The purpose, function, and nonprofit status of this organization and the exempt status for federal income tax purposes:
☐ Has Not Changed During Preceding 12 Months
☐ Has Changed During Preceding 12 Months (Publisher must submit explanation of change with this statement)

PS Form 3526, September 2007 (Page 1 of 3 (Instructions Page 3)) PSN 7530-01-000-9931 PRIVACY NOTICE: See our Privacy policy in www.usps.com

---

13. Publication Title	14. Issue Date for Circulation Data Below
Magnetic Resonance Imaging Clinics of North America	May 2010

15. Extent and Nature of Circulation		Average No. Copies Each Issue During Preceding 12 Months	No. Copies of Single Issue Published Nearest to Filing Date
a. Total Number of Copies (Net press run)		3402	3200
b. Paid Circulation (By Mail and Outside the Mail)	(1) Mailed Outside-County Paid Subscriptions Stated on PS Form 3541. (Include paid distribution above nominal rate, advertiser's proof copies, and exchange copies)	1616	1544
	(2) Mailed In-County Paid Subscriptions Stated on PS Form 3541 (Include paid distribution above nominal rate, advertiser's proof copies, and exchange copies)		
	(3) Paid Distribution Outside the Mails Including Sales Through Dealers and Carriers, Street Vendors, Counter Sales, and Other Paid Distribution Outside USPS®	497	522
	(4) Paid Distribution by Other Classes Mailed Through the USPS (e.g. First-Class Mail®)		
c. Total Paid Distribution (Sum of 15b (1), (2), (3), and (4)) ▸		2113	2066
d. Free or Nominal Rate Distribution (By Mail and Outside the Mail)	(1) Free or Nominal Rate Outside-County Copies Included on PS Form 3541	109	70
	(2) Free or Nominal Rate In-County Copies Included on PS Form 3541		
	(3) Free or Nominal Rate Copies Mailed at Other Classes Through the USPS (e.g. First-Class Mail)		
	(4) Free or Nominal Rate Distribution Outside the Mail (Carriers or other means)	109	70
e. Total Free or Nominal Rate Distribution (Sum of 15d (1), (2), (3) and (4)) ▸		2222	2136
f. Total Distribution (Sum of 15c and 15e) ▸		1180	1064
g. Copies not Distributed (See instructions to publishers #4 (page 83)) ▸		3402	3200
h. Total (Sum of 15f and g) ▸			
i. Percent Paid (15c divided by 15f times 100) ▸		95.09%	96.72%

16. Publication of Statement of Ownership

If the publication is a general publication, publication of this statement is required. Will be printed in the **November 2010** issue of this publication. ☐ Publication not required.

17. Signature and Title of Editor, Publisher, Business Manager, or Owner

Stephen R. Bushing
Stephen R. Bushing – Fulfillment/Inventory Specialist

Date
September 15, 2010

I certify that all information furnished on this form is true and complete. I understand that anyone who furnishes false or misleading information on this form or who omits material or information requested on the form may be subject to criminal sanctions (including fines and imprisonment) and/or civil sanctions (including civil penalties).

PS Form 3526, September 2007 (Page 2 of 3)

Moving?

Make sure your subscription moves with you!

To notify us of your new address, find your **Clinics Account Number** (located on your mailing label above your name), and contact customer service at:

Email: journalscustomerservice-usa@elsevier.com

800-654-2452 (subscribers in the U.S. & Canada)
314-447-8871 (subscribers outside of the U.S. & Canada)

Fax number: 314-447-8029

Elsevier Health Sciences Division
Subscription Customer Service
3251 Riverport Lane
Maryland Heights, MO 63043

*To ensure uninterrupted delivery of your subscription, please notify us at least 4 weeks in advance of move.

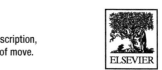
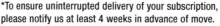

Printed and bound by CPI Group (UK) Ltd, Croydon, CR0 4YY

03/10/2024

01040356-0015